Essential
exercise

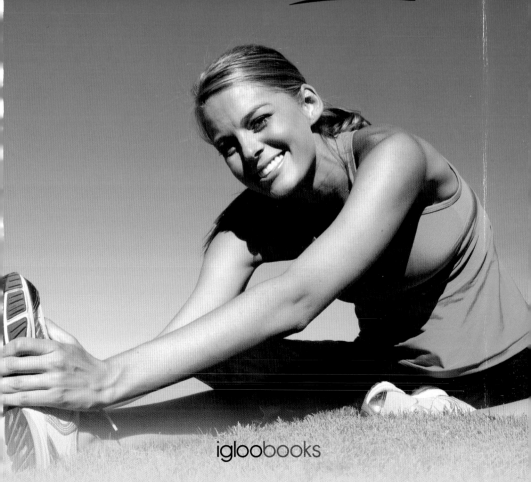

igloobooks

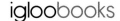

Published in 2014
by Igloo Books Ltd
Cottage Farm
Sywell
NN6 0BJ
www.igloobooks.com

FIR003 0514
2 4 6 8 10 9 7 5 3 1
ISBN 978-1-78343-466-4

Produced by Calcium Creative Ltd
Written by Jasmine Brooke
Consultant: Sandra Farnell

The following images are courtesy of Shutterstock
4, 5, 6, 10, 13, 18, 19, 20, 21 (main), 22, 25, 27, 31,
75, 76, 80, 87, 92, 96, 97
www.shutterstock.com

The following images are courtesy of Dreamstime
7, 8, 21 (bl), 28, 29, 30 (br), 32, 33, 39, 40, 43, 44, 47, 53,
62, 73, 103, 104, 105, 107, 109, 110, 111, 112, 113
www.dreamstime.com

Printed and manufactured in China

CONTENTS

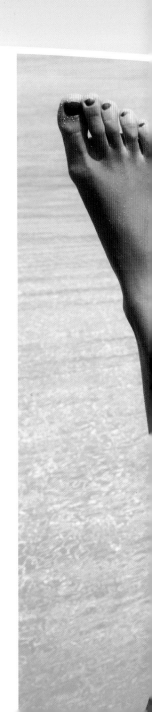

Essential exercise

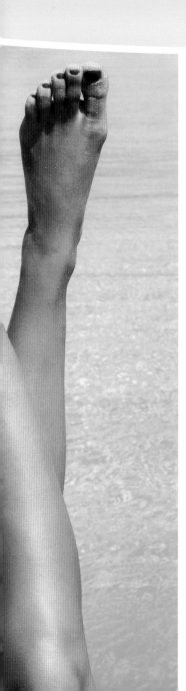

THE UPPER BODY

COUNTDOWN TO FITNESS

GLOSSARY
INDEX

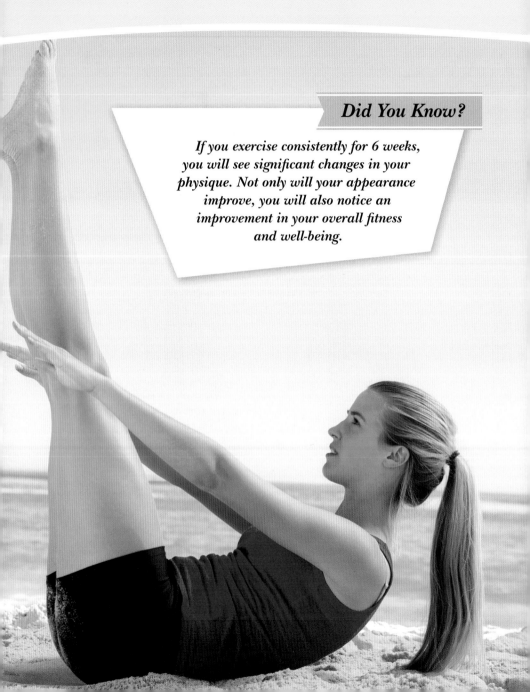

Did You Know?

If you exercise consistently for 6 weeks, you will see significant changes in your physique. Not only will your appearance improve, you will also notice an improvement in your overall fitness and well-being.

GET FIT FOR LIFE

Many people find the idea of getting in shape daunting and are often unsure about how to begin. There are no secrets to slimming, but with a little hard work and persistence, you can achieve great health in no time.

With a mixture of cardiovascular exercise and strength training, it is possible to lose body fat, condition your muscles and transform your body shape. This book explains how exercise can change your body, the many health benefits you will receive from fitness (as well as the aesthetic benefits) and how to incorporate a regular training programme within your life.

You'll learn how different exercises affect your body and how to target specific areas, as well as building a complete programme that will meet your individual needs and concerns. Whatever your starting body shape and size, regular exercise will help you to control your weight, sculpt and shape your body, lift your mood, as well as enable you to gain a sense of well-being and confidence.

Discover how working out and improving your fitness levels can be fun, rewarding and exciting. So let's get fit for life!

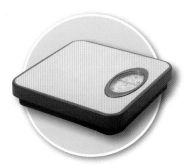

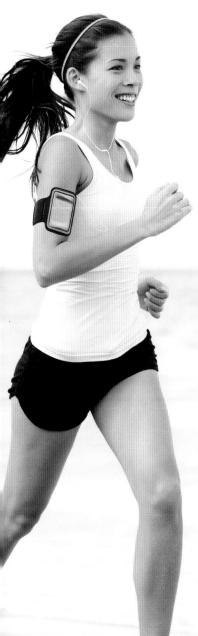

HOW TO USE THIS BOOK

Before you begin to plan your exercise regimen, take a look at the following information to help you get the most out of your fitness plan.

Getting in shape for life is a two-fold programme. The best way to shape up quickly and effectively is to combine a cardio fitness programme with a strength training routine. By utilising both exercise forms, you'll burn fat more quickly whilst shaping and toning your muscles. This book will show you how cardio and strength training exercises work, the benefits of both forms of exercise and how you can build your own routines.

1. Your Goals and Cardio Work

In the first section, we'll take a look at your goals so you can best determine the type of programme that is going to work for you. This section will also explain any equipment you may need and the best clothing to wear.

2. Strength Training Exercises

In the second section of this book, we'll examine strength training work in more detail. This section explains which muscle groups are important to train and how to train them. With clear, easy-to-follow step-by-step exercises, we'll guide you through each part of the body and how to train it to maximum effect. This section also contains some frequently asked questions to help you with any queries.

3. Your 6-Week Plan

In the final section of the book, we'll look at how you can create your own tailor-made, 6-week programme to get you in shape for summer.

This section explains how to plan your fitness regimen so that you will be in the best possible shape!

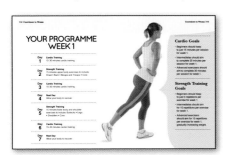

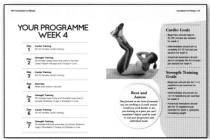

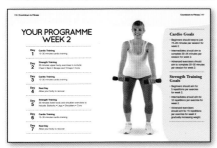

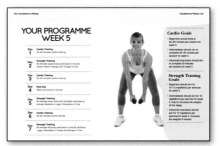

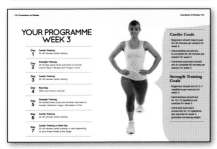

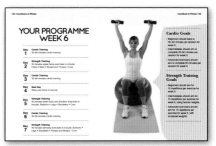

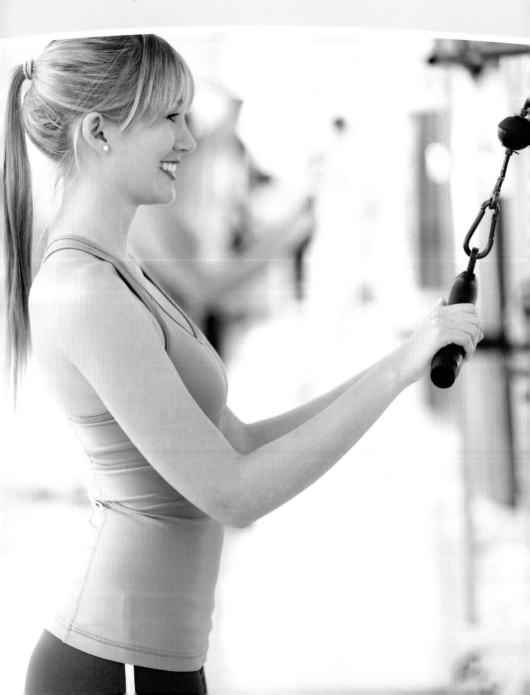

GOALS AND PLANNING

Setting goals and planning how to achieve them is key to getting in shape. The following section will explain how you can assess your individual fitness needs with an exercise regimen that is fun and realistically attainable.

If your aim is to get in shape for life, the likelihood is that you wish to improve your muscle tone and may wish to lose body fat, too. You may be a novice to exercise and in need of a beginner's programme to start exercising and shaping up. You may be a regular exerciser whose fitness regimen is too repetitive and no longer delivering results. Whatever your starting point, the key to any body-shaping programme is assessing your own individual needs and goals. Use the following section to choose your cardio exercise and plan your routine.

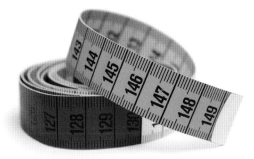

Body Fat

Excess body fat is an issue that affects many women and a number of men, too. Carrying too much body fat obscures the muscles of the body, can make the physique look unsightly, and is also uncomfortable. Carrying too much extra fat not only affects a person's appearance, it can be damaging to their health. Maintaining an optimum, healthy weight is a goal that can be achieved by everyone, with the right information and support.

Losing Body Fat

The most effective way to lose excess body fat is through cardiovascular exercise. This is a form of exercise in which your heart rate is raised, thereby increasing the flow of blood around your body. Cardiovascular exercise raises your metabolic rate during the time you exercise; it can also help to keep your metabolic rate higher after exercise, too. A higher metabolic rate burns more calories. This, combined with a sensible eating programme, means burning more body fat.

Cardiovascular Exercise

Cardiovascular exercise comes in many forms, from running and cycling through to swimming, aerobic classes and walking. The intensity at which you exercise during cardiovascular training has a bearing on the number of calories you will burn. Intense cardiovascular exercise will result in a greater calorie burn. However, the key to any cardiovascular workout is regularity – ensuring that you train regularly is more beneficial than carrying out an extremely intensive cardio session at the start of your programme and then being unable to sustain it. It is best to build up intensity at a rate that suits your body and your individual fitness levels.

Calorie Burning

On page 17, you will find a guide that shows the approximate number of calories burned during 30 minutes of sustained cardiovascular exercise. You can use the guide to help you build a cardio programme to lose body fat.

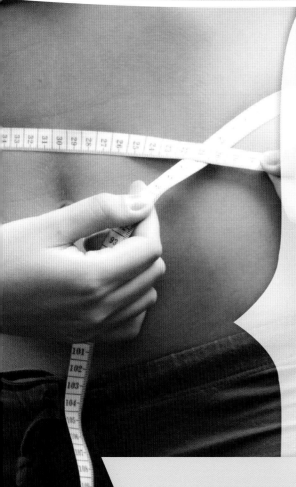

Assessing Body Fat

The easiest way to assess if you are carrying excess body fat is to carry out a Body Mass Index (BMI) analysis. A BMI analysis calculates whether you are carrying excess weight, or body fat, using your height and weight measurements. You can find a BMI calculator on the Internet to help you assess your weight. Below is a guide to help you work out if your ratio is within the healthy range:

Underweight: 18.5

Optimum Weight: 18.5–24.9

Overweight: 25.0–29.0

Obese: 30.0 +

Did You Know?

If you strength train regularly, you may find that your weight increases. Try to avoid becoming obsessive about how much you weigh. Remember that muscle weighs more than fat, so focus on a reduction of body fat rather than a reduction of weight.

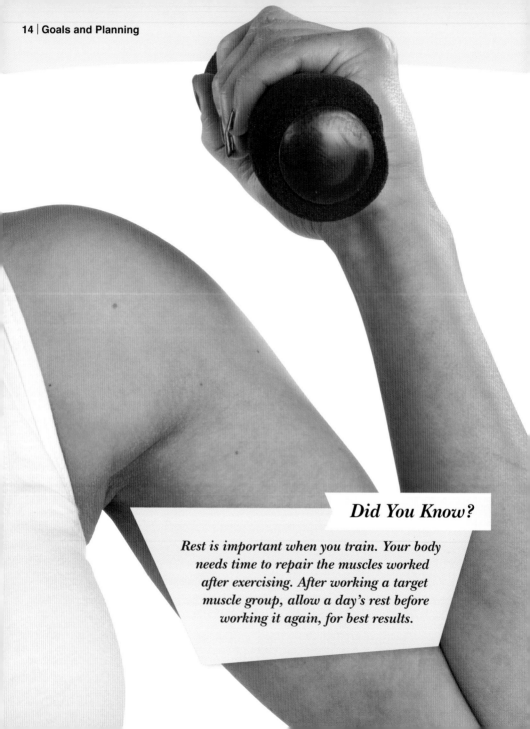

Did You Know?

Rest is important when you train. Your body needs time to repair the muscles worked after exercising. After working a target muscle group, allow a day's rest before working it again, for best results.

Muscle Tone

Along with concerns about excess body fat, many people are also worried that they are weak and their muscles lack shape and definition. Often referred to as 'flabby', unexercised muscles do not enhance anyone's physique. Muscles need to be exercised in order to maintain their tone. An under-exercised muscle will lose its 'mass' and weaken, thereby becoming loose and unshapely. Along with cardiovascular exercise, weight bearing, or strength training, exercise should form a key part of any fitness routine.

Strength Training and Health

Strength training exercise is essential to overall health. Strong muscles help support and protect the skeletal frame. Increased muscle mass also raises the body's resting metabolic rate, which means it will burn a greater number of calories even when not exercising.

Weight Bearing Exercise

Any form of weight bearing exercise will help build muscle mass. Weight bearing exercise includes the use of weights such as dumbbells, kettlebells and barbells, as well as resistance equipment such as resistance bands, and your own body weight. There are many exercises you can do to improve muscle tone using the weight of your body alone.

Targeting Concerns

The beauty of weight bearing exercise is that it is possible to target individual muscle groups and single them out for maximum results. For example, if you are concerned about the muscle tone of the back of your arms (the tricep muscle), you can carry out exercises to target this muscle alone. Likewise, if you wish to improve the muscle tone of your legs and buttocks, there are targeted exercises you can do to work these areas effectively.

Tailor-made Exercise

The key to strength training is to focus on the areas of concern and improve them with consistent exercise. Your programme can be altered and tailored to adapt to your changing needs. For example, if you feel you are overtraining a muscle and becoming disproportioned, you can simply lighten your weights and reduce your number of repetitions. Strength training is wonderfully easy to control and a fabulous way to refine your contours.

Cardio Boost

Cardiovascular exercise has endless benefits. It burns calories during exercise and boosts your metabolism post-exercise. It reduces cellulite, helps improve muscle tone and raises your mood by increasing the endorphin levels in your body.

Burning Fat

Cardiovascular training is simply one of the best ways to burn fat and lose weight. Any exercise that raises your heart rate is cardiovascular exercise. The guide on page 17 offers a range of cardio activities you could incorporate in your fitness routine, along with the approximate number of calories you will burn during 30 minutes of sustained activity.

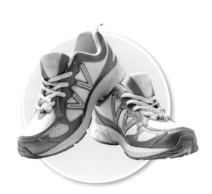

Mix it Up

To get the most from your cardio programme, choose activities you enjoy but also try to vary the activities. Cross-training, or using a mixture of exercise forms, is one of the best ways to ensure you fully train your body and thereby achieve optimum results. Mixing up your choice of exercise also helps to keep your interest levels up and avoid boredom.

How Often to Exercise

As a general guide, aim to carry out your cardio training sessions three to five times a week. The more often you exercise, the quicker you will see results.

Did You Know?

Combining cardiovascular exercise with gentle exercise that focuses on stretching the muscles, such as yoga or pilates, can be very beneficial. Concentrated stretching can help to ease tired, aching muscles and can also induce a feeling of calm.

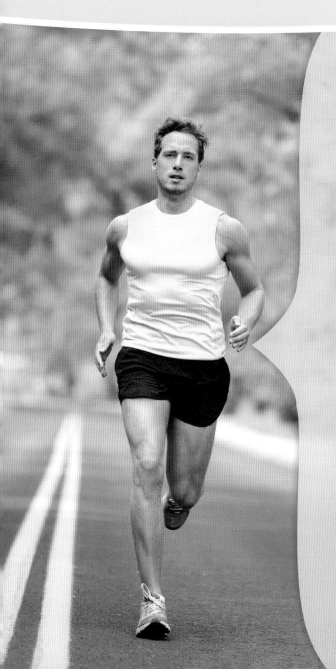

Calorie Burning Guide

During a 30-minute exercise session, you can expect to burn the following calories:

Running 360 calories

Cycling 340 calories

Swimming 250 calories

Cardio exercise class 340 calories

Cardio Benefits

- **Reduced body fat**
- **Improved fitness levels**
- **Improved circulation**
- **Increased muscle tone**
- **Improved skin tone**
- **Mood lift**

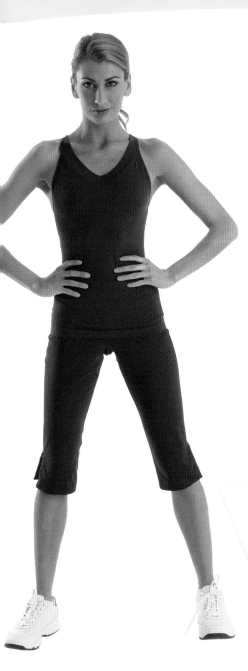

Cardio Equipment

Once you have established the cardio exercises you are going to incorporate into your exercise programme, you'll need to ensure you have the right equipment to carry them out. At a most basic level, the only key pieces of equipment you really require are a good pair of trainers or running shoes and comfortable exercise clothes. Below are some guidelines about what equipment to choose to get your exercise programme off to the best possible start.

Running

To run, all that is required are running shorts, trousers or leggings, a t-shirt and a sweat-top for warming up, and for women, a good sports bra. If you are running in cold weather, wear a warm hat and gloves. The key piece of equipment for any runner is a good pair of running shoes. This is one area where you should not cut corners in terms of investment. Good running shoes will help you avoid injury by properly supporting your feet, ankles and legs as you run. There are many specialist running shops that can help you choose a good pair of shoes if you need further help.

Did You Know?

If you wish to attend yoga or pilates classes, try to wear loose, comfortable clothing. Tight, restrictive clothing will limit your range of movement.

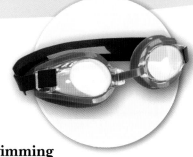

Walking

As with running, the best investment for this form of exercise is a good pair of shoes or walking boots. Choose a quality pair of shoes for foot, ankle and leg support. Loose, comfortable and weather-appropriate clothing will make walks more enjoyable, too.

Cycling

If you are new to cycling and would like to try it before making an investment in a bike, you may want to borrow or hire one first. Also assess if you are likely to be cycling mainly on the road, or if you prefer the idea of off-road cycling and mountain-biking. The two types of bikes needed for both activities are very different – road bikes are lighter, slimmer bikes designed to travel at speed. Mountain bikes are sturdier bikes, designed for rough terrain. You will also need a helmet, sunglasses and possibly gloves, for hand protection and improved handle grip.

Swimming

If you don't already own one, invest in a comfortable swimsuit in which you can easily swim. Goggles will prevent chlorine getting in the eyes, and help you see where you are going so you can swim more effectively. You can also consider a swimming hat and plugs for the ears and nose if incoming water puts you off your stroke!

Exercise Classes

A good pair of trainers is a must for a class activity, along with comfortable clothing. There are many forms of exercise clothes now available that wick sweat away from the body during exercise, helping to keep you drier during workouts.

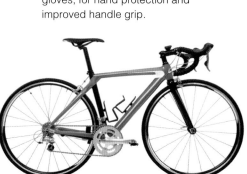

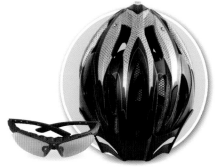

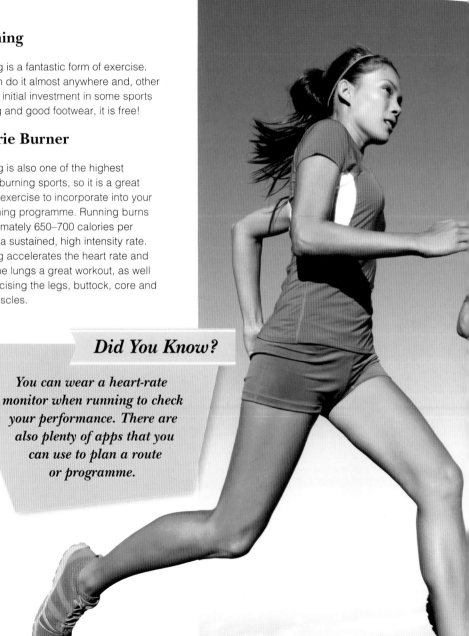

Running

Running is a fantastic form of exercise. You can do it almost anywhere and, other than an initial investment in some sports clothing and good footwear, it is free!

Calorie Burner

Running is also one of the highest calorie burning sports, so it is a great form of exercise to incorporate into your fat-burning programme. Running burns approximately 650–700 calories per hour at a sustained, high intensity rate. Running accelerates the heart rate and gives the lungs a great workout, as well as exercising the legs, buttock, core and arm muscles.

Did You Know?

You can wear a heart-rate monitor when running to check your performance. There are also plenty of apps that you can use to plan a route or programme.

Long or Short

Running can be adapted into either a long-distance activity or a short, intense workout. Some people find they do not have the time to run for long periods of time, so prefer to concentrate on short, intense runs that work the body to maximum effect in a minimal time period. Others prefer to run for greater distances, over a longer period of time, but at a reduced intensity. Whatever your preferences and requirements, you can adapt your running routine to suit your needs.

Run Anywhere

Running can be carried out almost anywhere. You can run on the pavement, if you live in a town or a city, or you can cross-country run if you prefer. Lots of people enjoy running alone, whilst others like to be part of a running group or club for added motivation.

Reasons to Run

A low-cost, accessible sport

No gym membership required!

Sociable or singular sport

Great calorie burner

Can be carried out almost anywhere

Running Benefits

- **Improved leg muscle tone**
- **Greater buttock muscle tone**
- **Improved stomach muscle and arm tone**
- **Increased fitness**
- **Improved circulation**
- **Mood lift and weight loss**

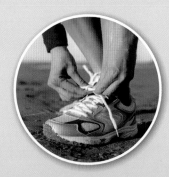

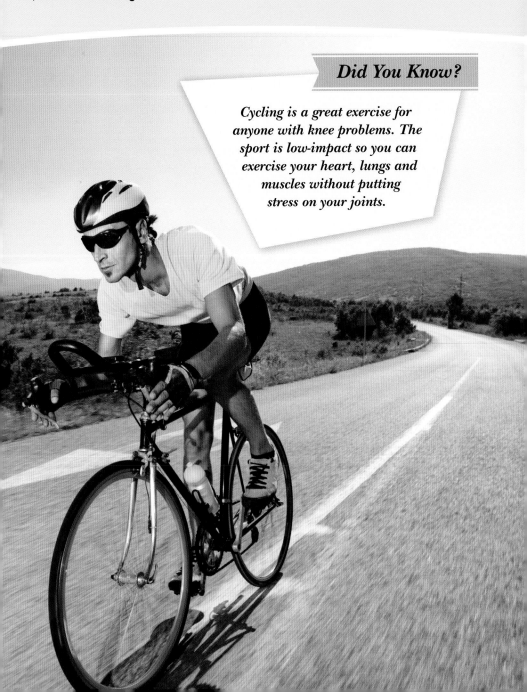

Did You Know?

Cycling is a great exercise for anyone with knee problems. The sport is low-impact so you can exercise your heart, lungs and muscles without putting stress on your joints.

Cycling

Like running, cycling is one of the most popular cardio exercises. Cycling is a fabulous lower-body workout. Regular cyclists have superb leg and buttock muscles because this exercise really concentrates on these muscle groups, working them to optimum results. You'll notice, if you cycle, that your buttock, thigh and calf muscles become a lot stronger, firmer and leaner as a result of regular cycling exercise.

Fat Burning

Cycling is also great calorie burner, burning up to approximately 600 calories per hour if carried out at a sustained, high intensity level.

On-road or Off-road

Cycling is an activity that can be enjoyed at ease, as long as you have access to good roads or tracks for mountain-biking. As discussed earlier, you can cycle on the road with a road bike, or off-road with a mountain bike. Mountain bikes are also fine for on-road cycling, although you will not achieve the speeds you will with a road bike. Hybrid bikes are a combination of road cycling bike features and mountain bike features, which can be used both on and off-road, with the correct tyres.

Single or Group Cycling

Like running, you can cycle alone as part of your fitness programme, or in a group if you prefer, for motivation and company.

Reasons to Cycle

No gym membership required!

Sociable or singular sport

Great calorie burner

Can be carried out almost anywhere

Cycling Benefits

- **Excellent for toning leg and buttock muscles**
- **Improved stomach muscle tone**
- **Increased fitness and weight loss**
- **Improved circulation**
- **Mood lift**

Swimming

Along with walking, swimming is one of the lowest-impact cardiovascular sports. Because the body is supported by water, there is little risk of any injury. For this reason, swimming is often a good choice for people unused to exercise but wishing to improve their fitness levels. It is also a good choice for people who are overweight – swimming can be a great way to get back into fitness, burn fat and improve muscle tone without putting stress on your joints.

Where to Swim

Many local sports facilities have swimming pools and offer times at which swimmers can lane-swim, or use the pool to exercise freely. Lane swimming is a great way to improve your fitness levels because you can swim consistently and uninterrupted. Bear in mind that if you try to swim during public swimming times, the pool can be crowded and swimming for fitness can be difficult. It is best to plan ahead to ensure you have space to swim without being disturbed.

Training Programmes

Many local leisure centres or pools offer swimming programmes that help you build up your fitness levels and technique week by week. Check out your facilities to see if you can find similar programmes to build into your exercise plan.

All-round Exercise

Swimming is great all-round exercise because it works almost every muscle group in the body. Swimming exercises the legs, core, back, arms and shoulder muscles – all at the same time. Swimming greatly improves muscle tone and is a superb cellulite reducer.

Fat Burning

Swimming does not burn as many calories per hour as running or cycling, however, an hour of moderately intense swimming still achieves good calorie-burning results at up to 500 calories per hour.

Did You Know?

Many people swim with their head above the water, but this can induce neck strain. Invest in a good pair of goggles and try to practise swimming face-down until you are comfortable with this position.

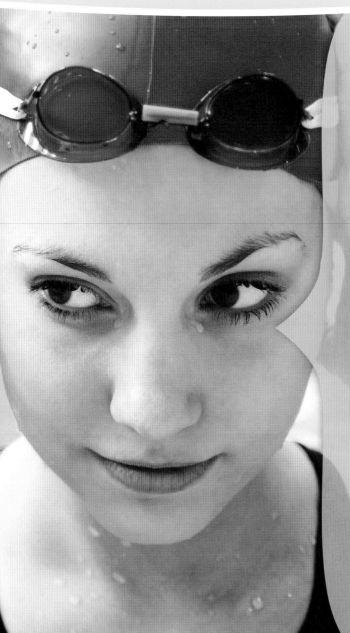

Reasons to Swim

Great exercise for beginners

Good for people carrying excess weight

Good all-round body conditioning

Swimming Benefits

- **Excellent for all-round muscle toning**
- **Increased fitness**
- **Low risk of injury**
- **Improved circulation**
- **Improved skin tone**
- **Mood lift and weight loss**

Exercise Classes

Exercise classes are a great way to begin exercising under supervision. Your local gym, or leisure centre, should have a programme of exercise classes that you can choose from.

Dance-based Classes

Most dance-based classes are cardiovascular, raising the heart rate and giving the lungs a good workout. They also work muscle groups such as the legs, core, and arms. Other dance-based classes include Zumba, hip hop and aerobic classes.

Circuit Training

Circuit training classes are popular with men and women alike. They usually involve high intensity intervals and short rests, which boosts metabolism and trains the heart and lungs, along with different muscles.

Body Combat

Martial arts classes, such as kickboxing, are great calorie burners. These high-intensity classes involve short, intense bursts of movement that work the body to maximum effect. Other combat-based classes, such as boxing classes, are also popular with both men and women and are great all-round cardiovascular workouts.

Sociable, Fun, Safe

Exercise classes can be a fun, sociable way to keep fit and help to sustain your interest levels during your fitness programme. A key advantage of attending exercise classes is motivation – a trained teacher can really help to motivate you and ensure you exercise to maximum effect. If you feel that an additional motivation boost could help you focus, or inject some interest into an existing exercise programme, then classes could be a great choice.

Did You Know?

Investigate stretch-based exercise classes such as yoga and pilates in your local area. Both forms of exercise will greatly improve your flexibility and help to alleviate stress.

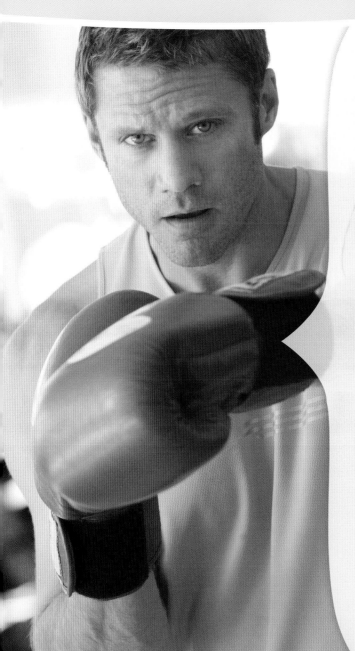

Reasons to Exercise in a Class

Great for beginners

Good for people in need of extra motivation

Sociable form of exercise

Exercise planned by trained supervisor

Class Benefits

- **Good for beginners unused to exercise**
- **Low risk of injury under supervision**
- **Improved circulation**
- **Improved skin tone**
- **Improved fitness**
- **Mood lift**

Strength Training

The benefits of training your muscles are enormous: with improved muscle density comes strength, a sleeker, more defined physique, even skin tone and higher metabolism.

Metabolic Burn

Not only does strength training improve the appearance of your muscles, it also helps to fire up your body's metabolic rate and therefore burn more fat. Gram for gram, muscle burns more calories than fat. If you increase your muscle mass, you greatly increase your fat-burning capacity. This means that even when you are not exercising, your body is still burning fat.

Sculpt and Tone

Strength, or weight, training is one of the best ways to sculpt your body. You can control which muscles you wish to build, the extent to which you build those muscles, and the overall shape you wish to achieve.

Women and Men

Many women are wrongly put off strength training because they believe they will build huge, bulky muscles. It is extremely difficult for most women to build huge muscle mass. You need to consume more calories than you burn to build bulk, and women do not have the levels of testosterone required to build muscles to the extent seen in men who weight and strength train.

Did You Know?

Strength training in front of a mirror is a great way to monitor your form. You can ensure you are performing each exercise correctly and adjust your weights if you notice any problems with technique.

However, for women, sustained strength training can achieve greatly improved strength and tone, and target specific areas that concern many women, such as the back of the arms, stomach, thighs and buttocks.

Strength Training for Men

For men, strength training can achieve a much improved physique, greatly increased muscle mass and tone, and a power-house metabolic rate that continuously burns fat.

Strength Training Benefits

- **Improved muscle tone**
- **Improved skin tone**
- **Better circulation**
- **Increased muscle strength**
- **Shapelier physique**

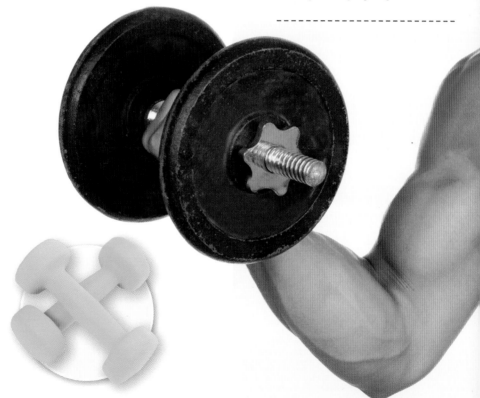

Muscle Tone Equipment

Using weights to increase muscle mass comes in a number of forms. Weights increase the intensity of an exercise performed to target a specific muscle group.

Dumbbells and Barbells

You can use dumbbells or barbells to work muscle groups. Dumbbells are hand-held weights (also known as free weights) that increase the intensity of exercises such as lunges, squats and bicep curls. Dumbbells with a foam outer covering are preferable for beginners because it is easier to grip the weight as you exercise. A barbell is a long bar with circular weights attached at each end. Like dumbbells, a barbell increases the intensity of any strength training exercise that is performed.

Dumbbells and barbells are a great investment if you are intending to exercise at home and do not wish to use, or do not have access to, a gym.

Resistance Bands

Like dumbbells and barbells, resistance bands are hand-held pieces of equipment that increase the intensity of a strength training exercise. Made of rubber or elastic components, the bands stretch and contract with the activity, thereby working the muscles used to carry out the exercise more effectively.

Resistance bands are another great, low-cost investment for a home exercise programme.

Own Body Weight

Strength training can be carried out without any exercise equipment at all. Simply using your own body weight, it is possible to train many muscles of the body, from the legs, buttocks and back to the arms, chest and shoulders. There are a number of exercises in the later sections of this book that explain how you can exercise using your body weight alone.

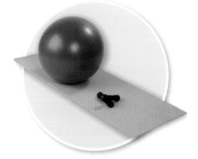

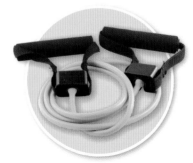

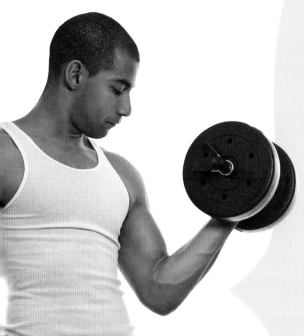

Reasons to Exercise

Ideal for a home exercise programme

Relatively low-cost initial investment

Easy to control amount of weight and repetition

Free Weights Benefits

- **Increased muscle mass**

- **Improved skin tone**

- **Equipment is portable**

Did You Know?

If you begin to find it easy to lift the weights you are currently using, don't be afraid to try heavier weights. Your muscles become used to exercise after a period of time, so you will need to challenge yourself again if you find that an exercise is becoming too easy.

Gyms

Most leisure facilities, or gyms, have strength training equipment. These may be static exercise machines that are used to target specific muscle groups as well as free weights.

Motivation and Help

Gyms can be a great place to exercise because many people find it motivating to workout with other people. Another advantage of gyms is that they are usually supervised, so if you are unsure about an exercise or would like more advice about your programme, you'll find somebody on hand to help.

Machines

Static machines are useful to beginners starting out on an exercise programme because they provide a rigid support for the body, which reduces the risk of injury. Static machines also allow the user to control the amount of weight they use to carry out the exercise, starting with very small, light weights and increasing, if desired, to heavy, intense weights.

Free Weights

Dumbbells are often available at most gyms. The range of hand-held weights at gyms is usually extensive and, for that reason, you'll find you can build a more advanced strength training programme than you might be able to at home.

Gym Training

Most gyms offer an induction programme, which explains to the user how to use the gym equipment. Gyms can also offer personalised exercise programmes, which can be a great incentive for beginners to exercise as well as a relatively cost-effective way of creating a personalised strength training programme to follow.

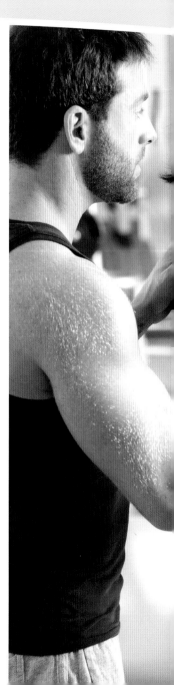

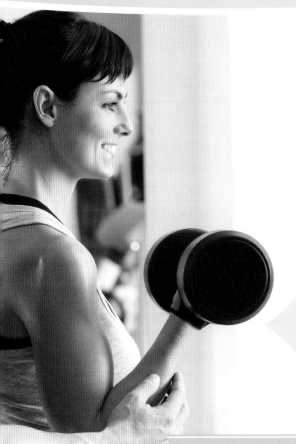

Reasons to Attend a Gym

Great environment in which to workout

Great scope for building up a more complete strength training programme

Expert advice on hand

Gym Benefits

- **Large range of equipment**
- **Exercise classes to suit all abilities**
- **Cardio workouts are also possible in gyms, along with strength training programmes**

Did You Know?

Gym staff are well-trained and able to help you with any queries or concerns you have. Don't be afraid to ask for help or advice when you use a gym.

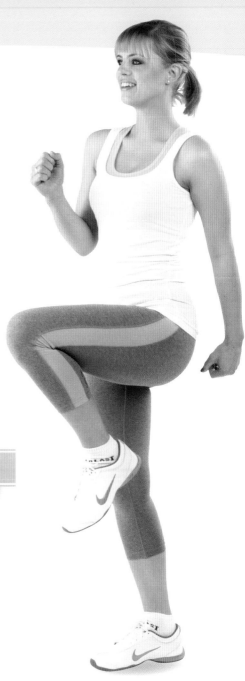

Warming Up

No exercise activity should begin without a thorough warm-up. A number of gentle stretches and movements are ideal, as they 'warm' the muscles, preparing the body for a more high-impact workout. If you begin to exercise without warming up your muscles, there is a risk that you could injure yourself during the activity. Warming up ensures that your muscles are ready to function properly.

Cardio Warm-up

A warm-up for cardiovascular exercise should include some light to brisk activity, such as walking or jogging on the spot. This will gradually raise the heart rate without shocking the body, and will utilise the muscles in preparation for the workout.

Did You Know?

You should feel your body becoming warmer and your breathing more laboured during your warm-up.

Strength Training Warm-up

A warm-up for strength training is also essential to avoid injury. The type of warm-up you carry out depends on the nature of the strength training you are going to do: be it a fast-paced routine with light weights, or a slower-paced routine using heavier weights.

Fast Workouts

Fast-paced, light repetition strength training exercise works the cardio system along with the muscles. If you intend to complete a lightweight, fast-paced strength training session, try to also include some cardio-based warm-up activities such as walking, light jogging, or star jumps to help prepare your heart and lungs for some vigorous activity. Also ensure you include some squats and large arm rotations in your warm-up to ensure your muscle groups are fully prepared for the exercise ahead.

Slow Workouts

If you intend to complete a slower, heavier-weight strength training session, you don't necessarily need to include a cardio-based warm-up. Although, in slow, heavyweight sessions, there is some strain on the heart and lungs – the focus is more intensely on particular muscle groups. Make sure you fully warm up the muscle groups you intend to work, such as the legs and buttocks with squats and lunges, and the upper body with some large arm rotations.

Cardio Warm-up Check List

☐ Start with gentle activity that raises the heart rate, such as jogging or fast-paced walking.

☐ Continue the warm-up for at least 5 minutes.

☐ Make sure your body is warm and your heart rate is raised before beginning your workout.

Strength Training Warm-up Check List

☐ Start with activity that gently raises the heart rate, such as jogging or fast-paced walking if preparing for a lightweight, fast-paced workout.

☐ Include large movements such as arm rotations and squats.

☐ Continue the warm-up for at least 5 minutes.

☐ Make sure your body is warm before beginning your workout.

Cooling Down

Not only is it very important to prepare your body for exercise with a warm-up, it is also equally important to 'cool down' the body post-workout. After a cardio workout, the heart rate is still high and needs to be gently taken back to a normal rate. Stopping a cardio workout suddenly, when you are at the peak of activity and the heart rate is high, can shock the body and make the transition to normal activity difficult. There is also the risk of muscle tear or strain after any cardio activity that does not include a cool-down and stretch.

When you have worked your muscles, they need to be slowly taken back to a more 'usual' state through gentle stretching. Stretching helps ease the muscles after an intense workout and thereby avoids the risk of injury.

Cardio Cool-down

To cool down after a cardio workout, spend 3–5 minutes walking or gently jogging to bring down your heart rate. Finish the cool-down with 5–10 minutes of gentle stretches to help relax the muscles by using the stretch steps shown in the photographs opposite.

Strength Training Cool-down

To cool down after a strength training workout, spend 5–10 minutes gently stretching the muscle groups you have worked by using the stretch steps shown in the photographs opposite.

Cardio Cool-down Check List

☐ Include activity that gently lowers the heart rate such as light jogging or walking.

☐ Complete the cool-down with 5–10 minutes of stretching.

Strength Training Cool-down Check List

☐ Concentrate on easing the muscles you have worked with 5–10 minutes of stretching.

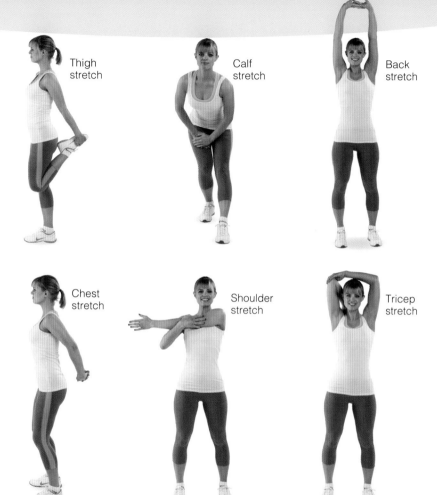

Thigh stretch

Calf stretch

Back stretch

Chest stretch

Shoulder stretch

Tricep stretch

Did You Know?

If you have worked a particular muscle group especially hard, you should take a few minutes longer to stretch that area to help return the muscles to their normal resting state.

YOUR RUNNING PROGRAMME

For all-round, superb cardio training and calorie burning, you can't beat running.

If you are a novice runner, you will need to begin your programme slowly. On the pages of your 6-week programme are options for beginners, intermediate runners and advanced runners. Start with the programme that currently best suits your ability, then build up to the more advanced timetables.

To Start Running

Warm up with gentle walking. Once your body is warm, increase your pace until you can feel your heart rate accelerate and your body temperature rise further. Try to swing your arms to help increase your heart rate. Take deeper, longer strides to warm up your legs. Continue for 5 minutes. Then begin your training programme.

How Do You Feel?

Assess how you feel as you carry out your programme and if you are finding it too easy, slowly increase the intensity of the exercise. If you are running on a treadmill, for example, increase the speed at which you are running. If you are running outdoors, try to increase the speed you run between landmarks, such as between lamp posts or trees, or simply increase your stride, to boost your cardio capacity.

Are You Training Hard Enough?

A good assessment of how hard you are training is to measure how you feel at the end of the faster run sections of the 6-week programme – if you feel out of breath and that you can't carry on during the accelerated running sections, you are working hard. If you feel you could happily carry on running for longer, reassess the effort you are putting in and consider running at a higher speed for these sections.

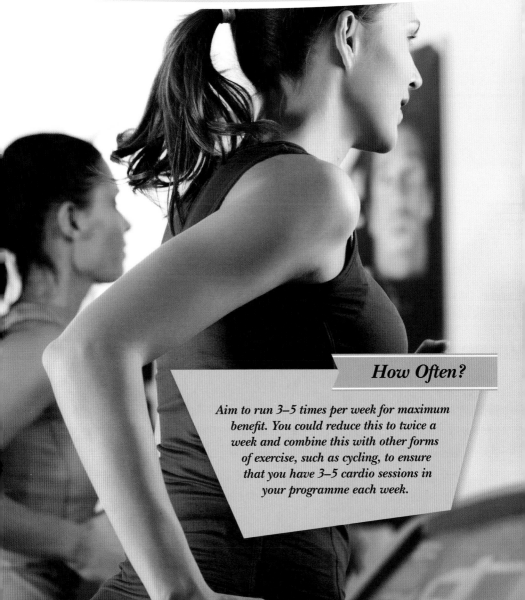

How Often?

Aim to run 3–5 times per week for maximum benefit. You could reduce this to twice a week and combine this with other forms of exercise, such as cycling, to ensure that you have 3–5 cardio sessions in your programme each week.

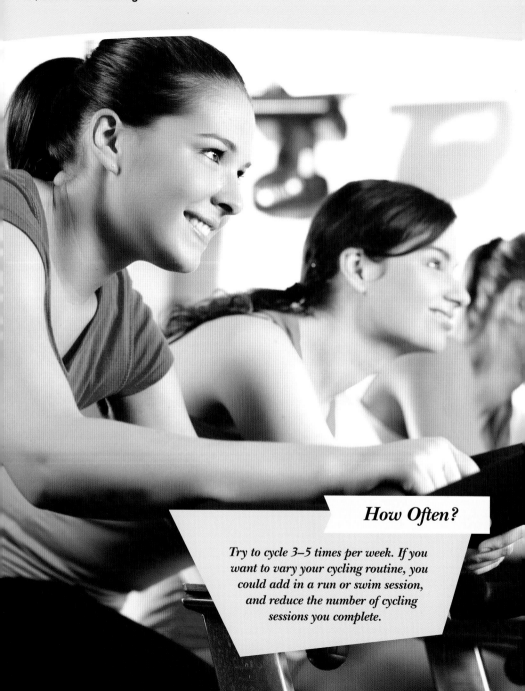

How Often?

Try to cycle 3–5 times per week. If you want to vary your cycling routine, you could add in a run or swim session, and reduce the number of cycling sessions you complete.

YOUR CYCLING PROGRAMME

Cycling is a great lower-body toning exercise that also works the cardio system with effective results.

For both experienced and beginner cyclists, consider planning a variety of routes to keep your levels of interest up. The same applies if you are intending to use your cycling programme in the gym – stationary gym bikes have plenty of varied cycle programmes that you can use to avoid becoming bored. On the 6-week programme pages are options for beginners, intermediate cyclists and advanced cyclists. Start with the programme that currently best suits your ability, then build up to the more advanced timetables.

Getting Started

Warm up with a gentle cycling pace, continue until you feel you are fully warmed up and ready to work harder. You'll need to get your leg muscles and heart and lungs fully warmed up in readiness for your workout. Adjust the gears on your bike to increase or reduce the intensity you are cycling at as required. Try to increase the intensity gradually for the first 5 minutes of cycling. When you are fully warmed up, begin your training programme.

Self-assessment

Don't forget to check how you feel as you work out – if you are finding that you are very out of breath and struggling, slow down and lower the gear level. If you feel that you could do more, increase the gear level and/or speed. If you are cycling on a bike in the gym, for example, increase the resistance at which you are cycling, or the speed. If you are cycling outdoors, try to increase the gear intensity to push yourself, and the speed at which you cycle at the same time. Alternatively, if you want to challenge yourself, then look out for hillier routes.

Hard or Easy?

To work out how hard you are training, measure how you feel at the end of the faster cycle sections of the 6-week programme – if you feel out of breath and that you can't carry on cycling any longer during the accelerated cycling sections, you are working hard. If you feel you could easily carry on cycling for longer, reassess the effort you are putting in and consider training at a higher speed and greater resistance for these sections.

YOUR SWIMMING PROGRAMME

Swimming is a superb, all-round exercise that works every part of the body with minimal stress.

Try to ensure you swim at a time that suits you and when the facilities you are using are not too busy to allow swimming for exercise. It is impossible to swim properly at times when the pool is full of people who just want to have fun rather than swim for fitness! Lane swimming sessions will allow you to swim lengths without obstruction. You can then concentrate on your technique and performance, rather than avoiding other people in the pool.

In the 6-week programme are options for beginners, intermediate swimmers and advanced swimmers. Start with the programme that currently best suits your ability, then build up to the more advanced timetables.

Begin to Swim

Warm up with a few gentle lengths of the pool – aim to swim slowly for around 5 minutes to make sure your body is used to the pool temperature and ready to work harder. Concentrate on breathing slowly and regularly with each stroke. Relax your shoulders as you swim. When you are warmed up, begin your programme.

How Does it Feel?

As with the running and cycling programmes, try to make an assessment of how hard you are swimming. Are you finding it very easy, or are you out of breath and exhausted? You can swim for longer with each programme if you want to increase your endurance. You can accelerate the speed at which you swim each length, and also reduce the number of slower-speed lengths in the 6-week programme, which will increase your cardio capacity.

Hard or Easy?

Don't forget to measure how you feel at the end of the faster swim sections of the 6-week programme – If you feel you could carry on swimming for longer, take another look at the effort you are putting in and consider training at a higher speed for these particular sections. If you feel out of breath and that you can't carry on swimming at the end of the accelerated swimming sections, you are working hard.

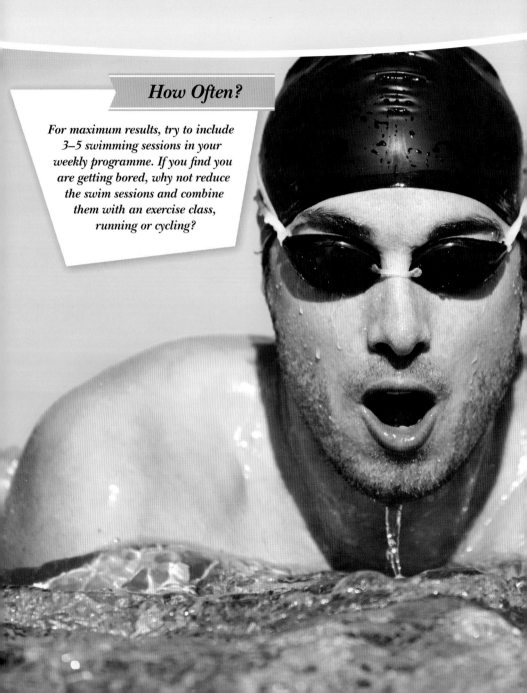

How Often?

For maximum results, try to include 3–5 swimming sessions in your weekly programme. If you find you are getting bored, why not reduce the swim sessions and combine them with an exercise class, running or cycling?

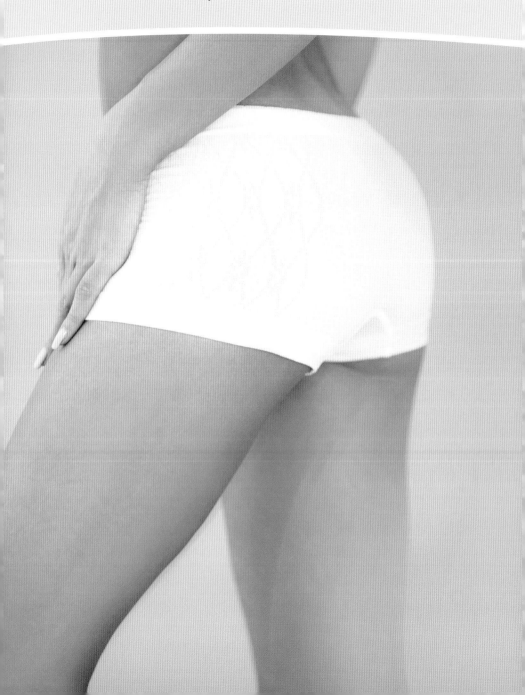

MUSCLE TONING FOR THE LOWER BODY

Toning your muscles is one of the most effective ways to restructure your body's contours. If you put in enough effort and concentration, you can see results in relatively short periods of time.

Strength training increases the size of your muscles, thereby making your body firmer and stronger in appearance. Increased muscle mass maximises your body's calorie-burning capacity, which helps you lose body fat, too. This increased metabolic rate, even when you are not training, is one of the key reasons why it is so important to combine a strength training regimen with a cardio programme for the best body-shaping results. The lower body has some large, powerful muscles which include the muscles of the buttocks and thighs. These sizeable muscles can withstand and respond well to intense training.

CORE

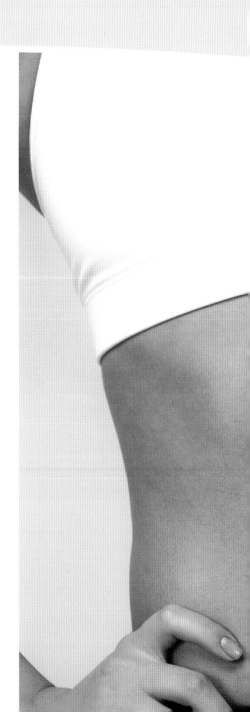

Core Exercises

There are four muscle groups in your abdominal area. The core muscles most commonly trained are the six-pack muscles. These are the muscles that run from your ribcage to your hipbones. The side muscles, also known as the 'obliques', are made up of both internal and external muscles. When trained properly, these muscles create the 'nipped in' waistline many women seek when shaping up. Lastly are the deeper abdominal muscles that are often not properly trained. It is important to train these muscles because they help you maintain proper posture and balance.

Body Fat and Abdominals

The stomach area can be difficult to flatten and shape unless combined with an effective cardio programme and a sensible eating plan. If body fat is reduced, it is possible to see the stomach muscles that you have worked so hard to create. With excess body fat, no matter how hard you work on your abdominals, it will be difficult to see results. A programme that targets body fat and increases muscle toning, achieves the best results in this area.

Technique and Control

When performing any of the stomach exercises on the following pages, aim to perform them slowly and concentrate on quality over quantity. It is better to start with a few repetitions, properly performed, than to try to perform multiple repetitions badly. Best results are achieved with concentrated training and good technique.

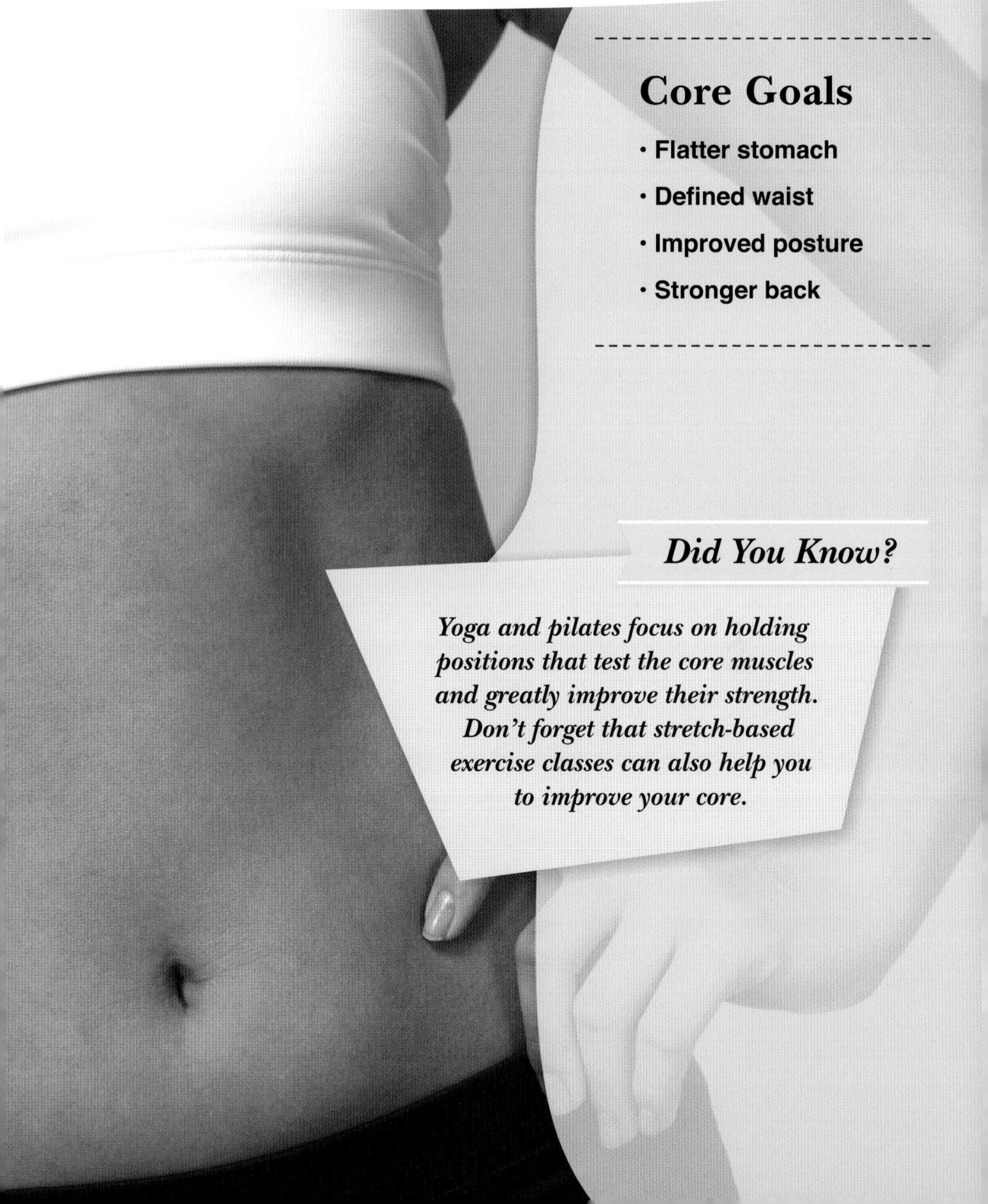

Core Goals

- **Flatter stomach**
- **Defined waist**
- **Improved posture**
- **Stronger back**

Did You Know?

Yoga and pilates focus on holding positions that test the core muscles and greatly improve their strength. Don't forget that stretch-based exercise classes can also help you to improve your core.

FOCUS: CORE

Crunches

- Lie with the fingers touching the temples and the legs curled in

- 'Crunch' by moving the knees towards the forehead and the forehead towards the knees

- Begin with one set of 20 crunches, increasing the number of sets

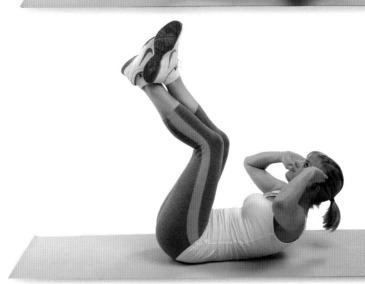

Bicycles

- Lie in the crunch position
- Pull the knee towards the opposite elbow and twist the elbow towards the knee
- Repeat on the opposite side, with 20 leg extensions in each set

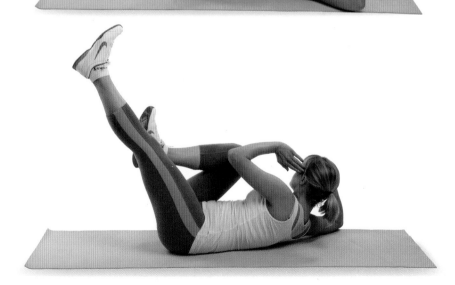

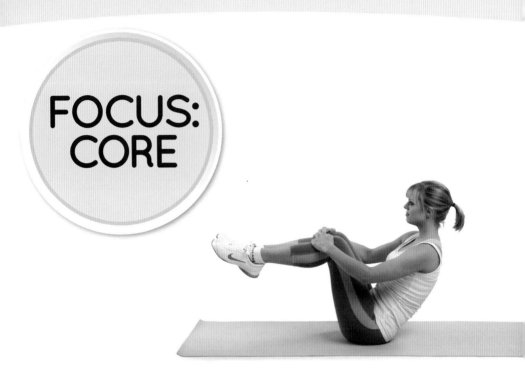

FOCUS: CORE

V Extension

- Sit with the hands grasping the knees and feet off the floor, calves parallel to the floor

- Leaning backwards, extend the arms to the side and extend the legs forward

- Return to the start and repeat the exercise with 20 extensions in each set

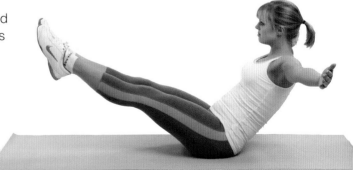

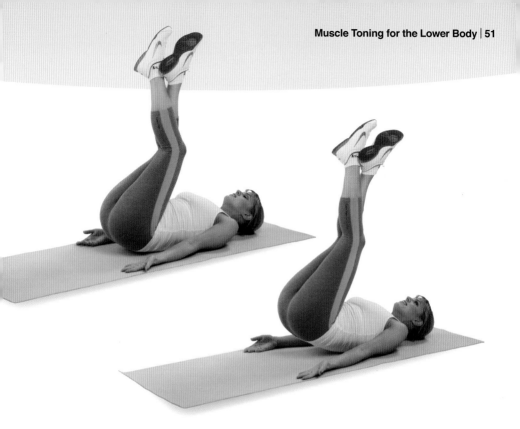

Lower Body Lifts

- Lie with the back flat to the ground, the arms extended by your side and the palms facing upwards

- Cross the legs in the air with feet flexed, facing the ceiling

- Extend the legs into the air, so that your bottom and lower back lifts off the floor. This should be a very small movement that uses the muscles of the lower stomach

LEGS

Leg Exercises

Toned, strong and shapely legs look great in summer wear, for instance, a dress or a pair of shorts. Many women are concerned with the shape of their legs, particularly the inner and outer thighs. Sculpting and toning this area can help reduce body fat and improve the texture of the skin, thus reducing any cellulite.

Thighs and Calves

The legs are made up of the large muscles of the thighs and the smaller muscles of the calves. Both cardio exercise, such as cycling, running and swimming, and the strength training exercises on the following pages will help to shape and firm the legs.

Exercise and Eating

As with all sculpting exercise, best results will be achieved when combined with a cardio programme and a sensible eating programme that keeps body fat within an optimum range.

Precision and Technique

For best results, aim to perform the exercises on the following pages with precision and concentration. It is best to begin with a few, well-performed repetitions, then increase these once you are confident with the exercises.

Did You Know?

If you work your legs hard during a strength, or cardio training session, you will need to ensure that you stretch fully afterwards to avoid injury. If your muscles remain tight after exercise, there is a risk that you'll be very sore in the next few days and may find it difficult to train again for a while.

Leg Goals

- Shapely legs
- Lower body strength
- Improve flexibility

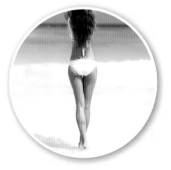

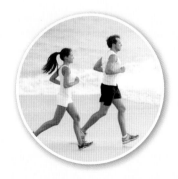

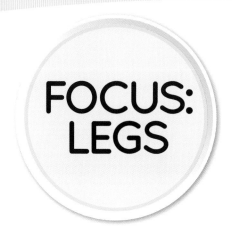

FOCUS: LEGS

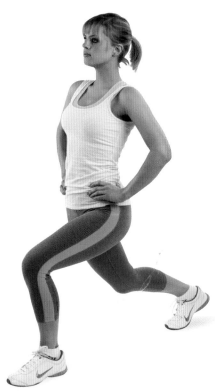

Lunges

- Stand with one leg bent in a lunge position, knee in line with the foot, the other leg extended backwards

- Put both hands on the hips for stability

- Complete your repetitions, then perform an equal number of repetitions with the other leg

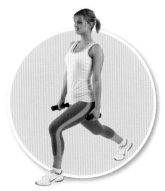

These exercises can also be performed using hand weights.

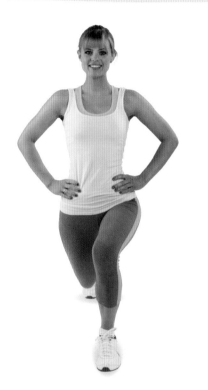 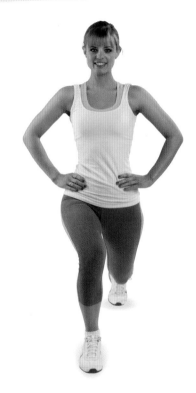

Standing Lunges

- Stand with both legs together, then lunge forward with one leg

- Return the leg to standing, then lunge forwards with the other leg

- Repeat an equal number of repetitions on both legs

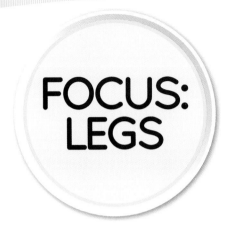

FOCUS: LEGS

Side Leg Lifts

- Lie on one side with the elbow on the ground and the head resting on the hand

- Position the feet and legs so they are stacked, one on top of the other

- Raise the upper leg into the air, ensuring the leg remains straight

- Lower the leg to the start position

- Repeat an equal number of times on both legs

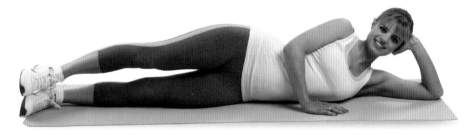

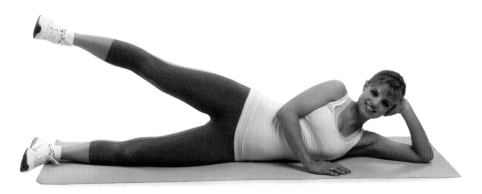

Leg Curls

- Lie on the back with the heels resting on an exercise ball, keeping the shoulders on the floor

- Curl and bring both knees in towards the chest so the ball is closer to the buttocks

- Extend legs and push the ball away

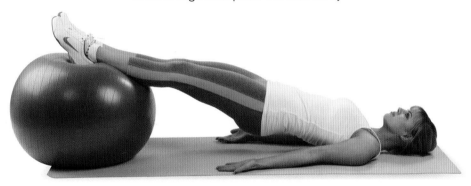

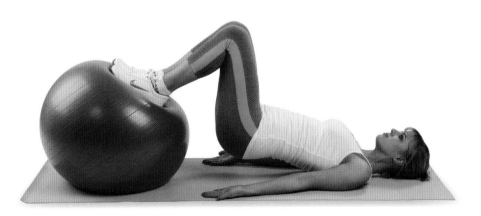

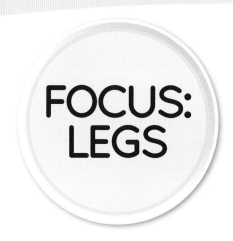

FOCUS: LEGS

Calf Raises

You can perform this exercise either on the ground or using a bench. You can hold onto the side of a chair or a wall for balance if you need to.

- Stand with the legs spaced shoulder-width apart

- Lift up onto the toes, feeling the stretch along the calf muscles

- Hold the position for 30 seconds, lower to the ground, and repeat

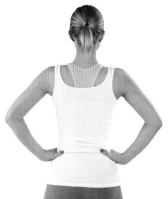

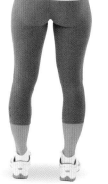

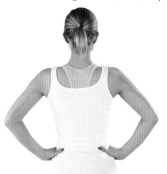

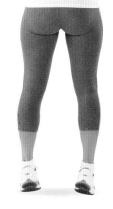

Inner Thigh Lifts

- Lie on one side, supporting your head with your arm, and stretch out one leg on the ground

- Bend the knee of the opposite leg and rest the foot on the ground, behind the knee of the stretched leg

- Raise your extended leg, keeping it straight, into the air. Feel the stretch along the inner thigh, then lower the leg to the ground

- Repeat an equal number of times on both legs

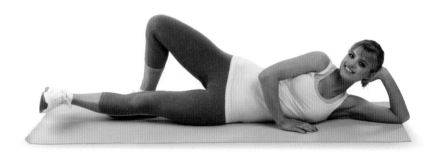

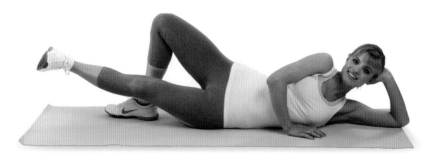

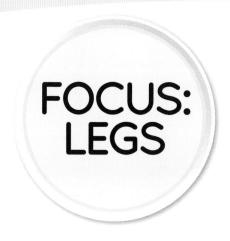

FOCUS: LEGS

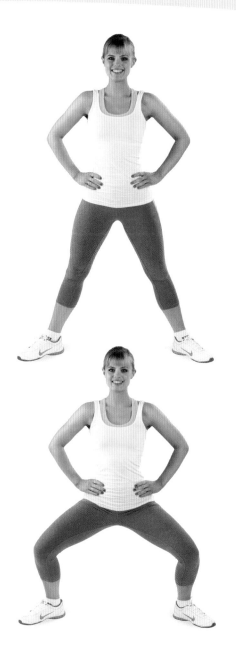

Pliés

- Stand with the feet hip-width apart, toes pointed outwards

- Bend the knees into a plié, feeling the stretch along the inner thighs and calves

- Return to standing and repeat

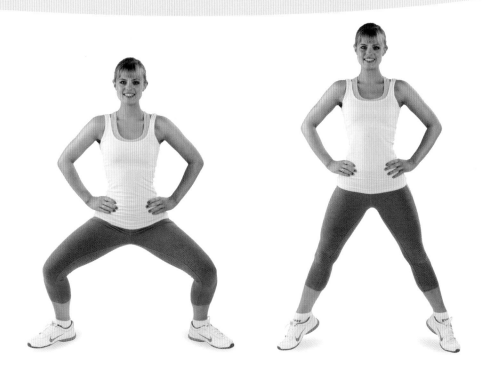

Pliés and Calf Lift

- Stand with the feet hip-width apart, toes pointed outwards

- Bend the knees into a plié, feeling the stretch along the inner thighs and calves

- Return to standing, then rise onto the toes, into a calf lift

- Return to standing and repeat

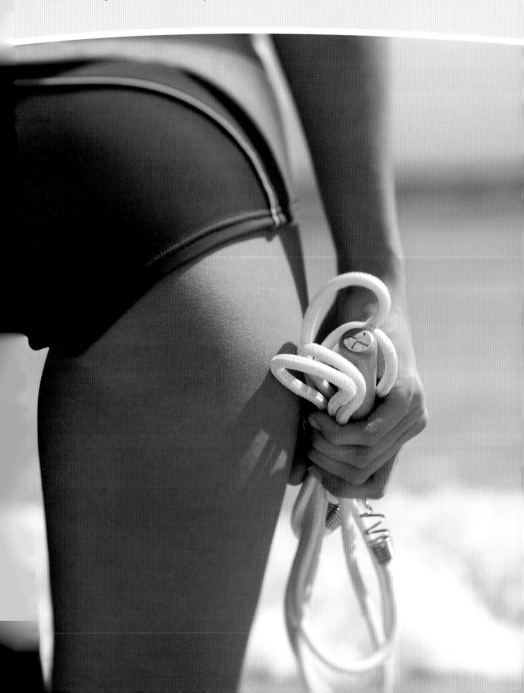

BOTTOM

Buttock Exercises

A tight, toned rear can be gained by concentrating on the gluteus maximus muscles, otherwise known as the 'glutes'. These are the largest muscles in the human body and, with concentrated work, can be built into a strong and fit shape.

Cardio Shaping

Cardio exercises such as running, and particularly cycling, are great for shaping the bottom. Strength training also focuses on this muscle group with great effect. Like the core muscles, strong buttock muscles are essential for maintaining overall fitness and mobility, so ensure that you incorporate the following exercises into your programme.

Working Hard

The large buttock muscles can be worked on intensively and can be exercised with heavier weights than smaller muscles, such as the shoulder muscles. Concentrate as you carry out the following exercises, focusing on the muscle group to make sure you perform the exercise with good technique. Aim for fewer repetitions to start with, building up to more as you become confident with the exercise.

Bottom Goals

- **Firm, toned rear**
- **Improved lower body strength**
- **Improved balance**

Did You Know?

There are some buttock exercises you can perform anywhere, anytime. For example, try clenching your buttock muscles when standing. You can also try some squats when watching television.

FOCUS:
BOTTOM

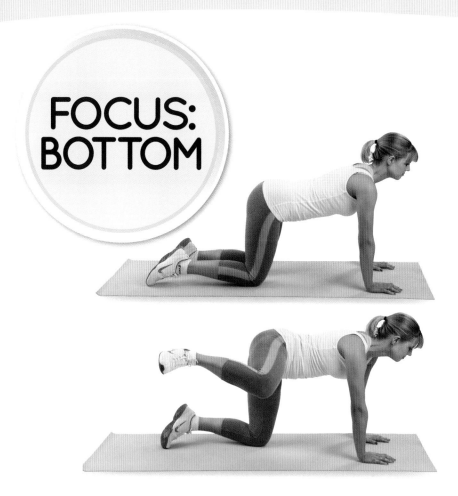

Side Leg Lifts

- Position yourself on all fours with a flat back

- Keeping the knee bent, lift one leg to the side, at hip height

- Hold the position for a couple of seconds

- Lower the knee to the starting position

- Repeat equally on both legs

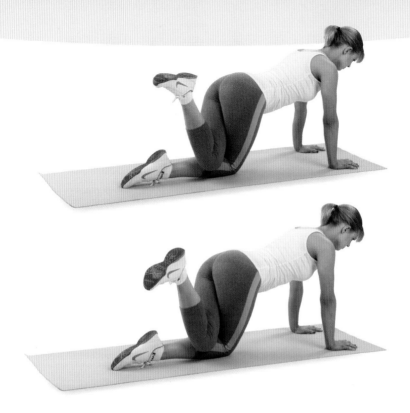

Leg Cross-overs

- Position yourself on all fours, with a flat back

- Keeping the knee bent, lift one leg and cross it over the opposite leg

- Dip the knee of the lifted leg into the knee of the stationary leg

- Feel the contraction in the buttock muscle

- Return to the starting position

- Repeat equally on both legs

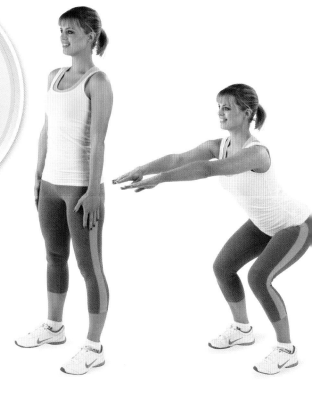

FOCUS: BOTTOM

Leg Squats

- Stand with the feet hip-width apart, toes facing forwards

- Push the bottom out and bend the knees into a squat position. Ensure the knees do not go over the toes

- Squat as deeply as possible and hold the position for 10 seconds

- Return to standing and repeat

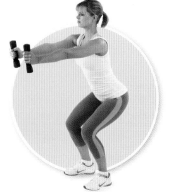

This exercise can also be performed using hand weights.

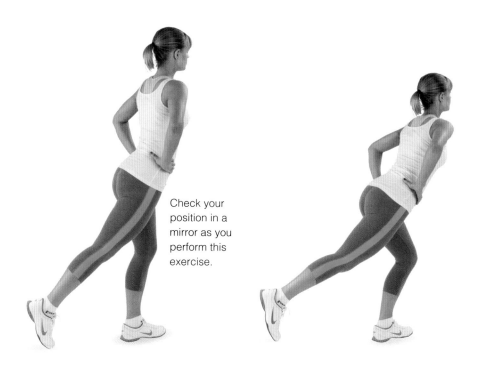

Check your position in a mirror as you perform this exercise.

Single Leg Squats

- Stand with the feet hip-width apart, toes facing forwards

- Bend the knee of one leg. Ensure the knees do not extend over the toes

- Extend the other leg behind you, foot raised off the floor

- Squat as deeply as possible onto the bent leg and hold the position for 10 seconds

- Return to standing

- Repeat equally on both legs

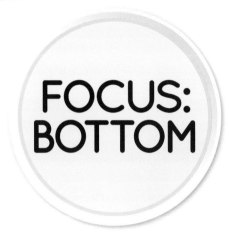

FOCUS: BOTTOM

Bridges

- Lie on the back with the feet flat on the floor, shoulder-width apart and arms by the sides

- Lift the bottom into the air, keeping the feet flat on the floor

- Clench the buttock muscles and hold the position for 30 seconds

- Return the bottom to the floor

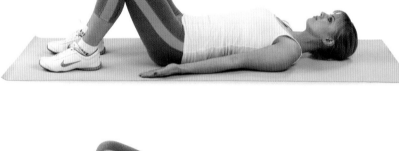

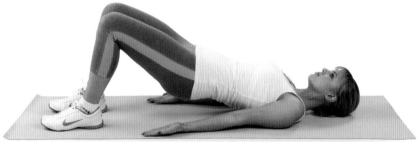

Bottom Raises

- Lie on the back with one foot resting on a surface, such as an exercise ball, the other foot raised in the air

- Lift the bottom away from the floor, clenching the buttock muscles

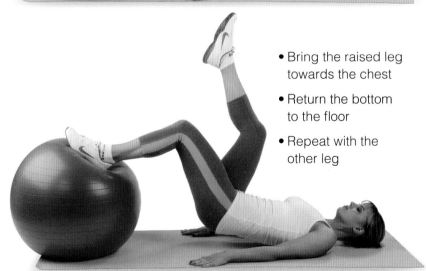

- Bring the raised leg towards the chest

- Return the bottom to the floor

- Repeat with the other leg

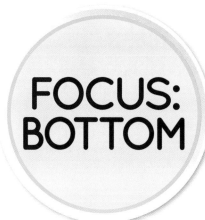

Rear Lifts

- Place the hands and knees on the floor, keeping the back straight

- Lift one leg to hip height, keeping the leg straight and the foot flexed. Hold the position for 30 seconds

- Return to the starting position

- Repeat equally on both legs

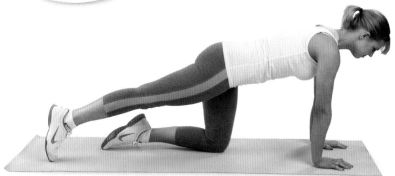

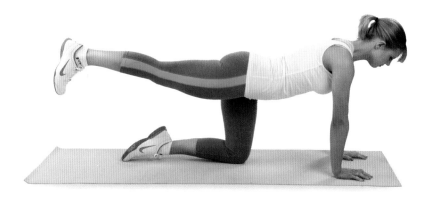

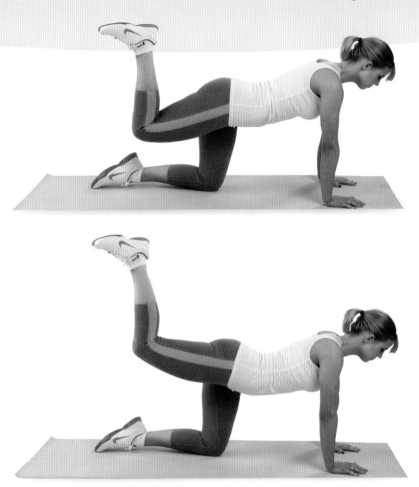

Rear Lifts and Raises

- Place the hands and knees on the floor, keeping the back straight

- Extend one leg backwards and bend at the knee 90 degrees

- Keep the foot flexed and lift the leg higher into the air, feeling the contraction of the buttock muscle

- Lower the leg to the starting position. Repeat equally on both legs

LOWER BODY Q&A

How do I avoid bulky muscles?

If you are female, this is highly unlikely! Unless you have extraordinarily high testosterone levels, it is impossible to build muscle mass to the equivalent of a male trainer.

I am carrying extra weight around my buttocks and thighs. Will strength training make me look even larger?

You may find as you start your training programme, that you go through a transition period in which you look slightly larger for a short period of time. Don't panic! This is simply a stage in which your body is building muscle, while reducing body fat. It takes time to lose weight sensibly, so persevere and you'll find that your fat levels reduce over time.

I have a knee injury. Can I strength train safely?

If you have concerns, always consult your doctor before beginning any exercise programme. If your doctor thinks it is safe for you to exercise, you should find that strength training helps to alleviate your problems. When you train your muscles, you also train the ligaments and tendons that support them and your skeletal system. This will, in turn, help to support areas of weakness in your body.

Can I reduce my muscle mass if I feel certain body parts are getting too big?

Yes! The beauty of strength training is that you can control it. Pay attention to the changes in your body and if you feel one area is becoming overdeveloped, simply reduce the time you spend training that muscle group. You can sculpt your body as desired, so focus on your physique and adjust your routine to suit your needs.

Can't I tone up my lower body through cardio alone?

Cardio exercise is great for reducing body fat and improving overall fitness and leg tone. However, to really develop the outline of your lower body, use strength training, too. Training with weight forces the large muscles of the lower body, such as the muscles of the buttocks, to increase in size and strength. This reshapes the outline of your lower body, making it appear firmer, leaner and stronger. You cannot achieve the same results through cardio exercise alone.

Will strength training improve my pear shaped body?

Absolutely. You should not only train your lower body, but also your upper body, so that eventually your physique will be more in proportion.

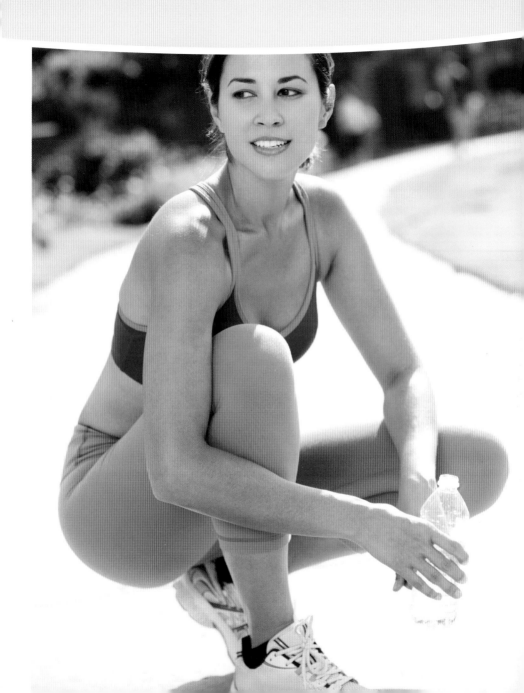

MUSCLE TONING FOR THE UPPER BODY

The upper body is made up of a variety of large and small muscles. The muscles of the back and chest are large muscles that can endure intense strength training with heavy weights. The muscles of the arms and shoulders are smaller, more compact muscles that need targeted training to obtain best results.

With focused training, it is possible to sculpt a toned and well-proportioned upper body. Men often focus on their upper body. However, many women ignore their upper body and concentrate solely on their legs and stomach. Don't make this mistake! A toned, lean and strong upper body can transform your body shape and dramatically improve your posture and overall health.

As with the strength training exercises already discussed for the lower body, ensure you combine your upper body programme with sensible eating and cardio work for best results. By maintaining an optimum body fat to muscle ratio, you'll be able to show off the results of your hard work.

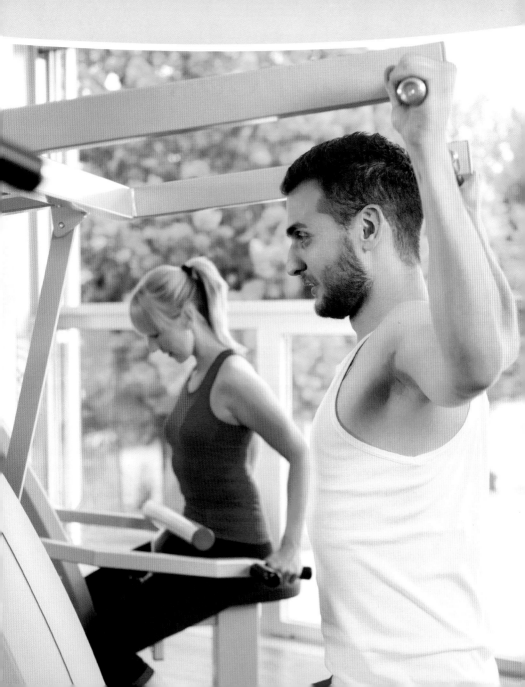

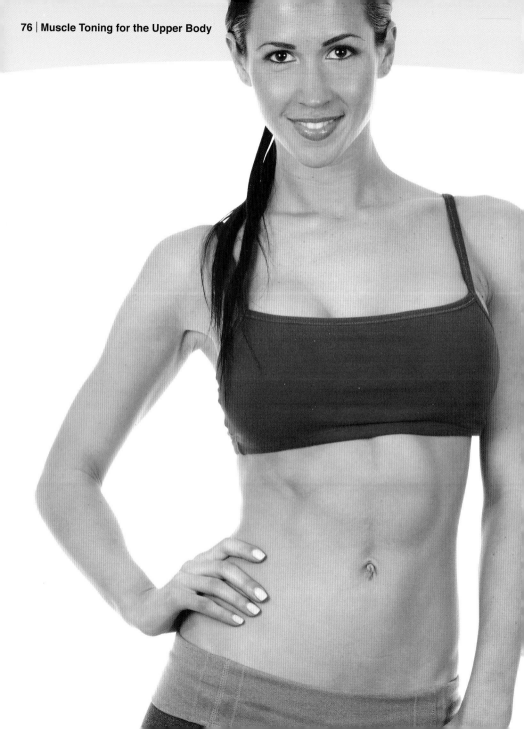

CHEST

Chest Exercises

Focusing on the muscles of the chest improves the overall shape of the upper body in both men and women. In men, it helps to build the pectoral muscles, better known as the 'pecs' and helps create a 'V-shape' physique. In women, working on the chest muscles helps to improve the bust line. Improving the muscle tone of the chest helps prevent sagging by keeping the bust high and firm.

Large Muscle Group

The chest muscles are a large muscle group and should be worked fairly intensively to achieve good results. Strong chest muscles, combined with a strong core and back, helps to create overall strength in the trunk of the body.

Building Up

Perform the following step-by-step exercises, focusing on good technique until you are accustomed to each movement. Once you are used to the exercises, build on repetition and, when you are ready, increase the weight to improve muscle strength.

Chest Goals

- **Improved appearance of bust in women**
- **Improved V-shape appearance in men**
- **Improved skin tone and elasticity**
- **Greater upper body strength**

Did You Know?

You should use heavier weights when training your chest muscles than you use when training smaller muscles, such as the shoulder muscles.

FOCUS: CHEST

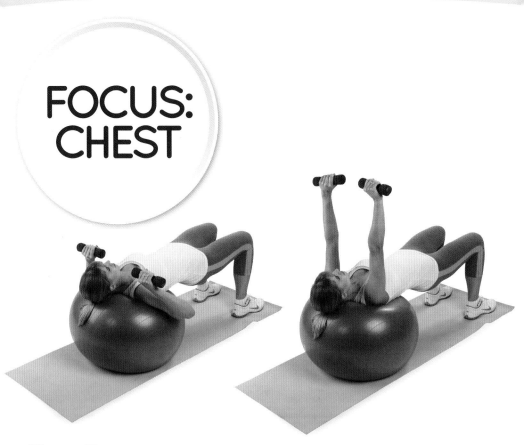

Chest Presses

You will need a bench, low table or a stability ball to perform this exercise. You will also need dumbbells, or other hand-held weights.

- Pick up the weights

- Lie on the bench or with the head, shoulders and upper back resting on an exercise ball

- Hold the weights at the side of the shoulders, with both arms bent

- Raise the weights into the air, directly above your shoulders

- Lower the weights back down to shoulder level, and repeat

Chest Flies

You will need a bench, low table or a stability ball to perform this exercise. You will also need dumbbells, or other hand-held weights.

- Pick up the weights

- Lie on the bench or with the head, shoulders and upper back resting on an exercise ball

- Hold the weights above the body, in line with the shoulders

- Extend the arms to the side of the body, until they are level with the shoulders

- Controlling the movement, raise the weights above the body and repeat

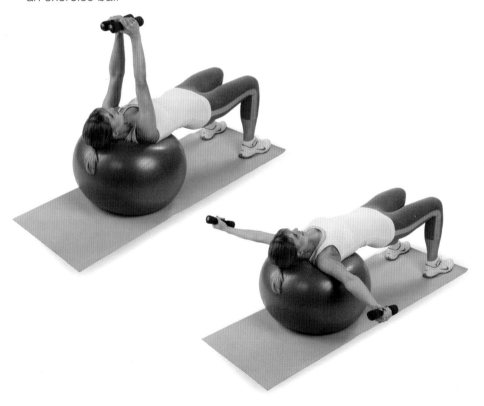

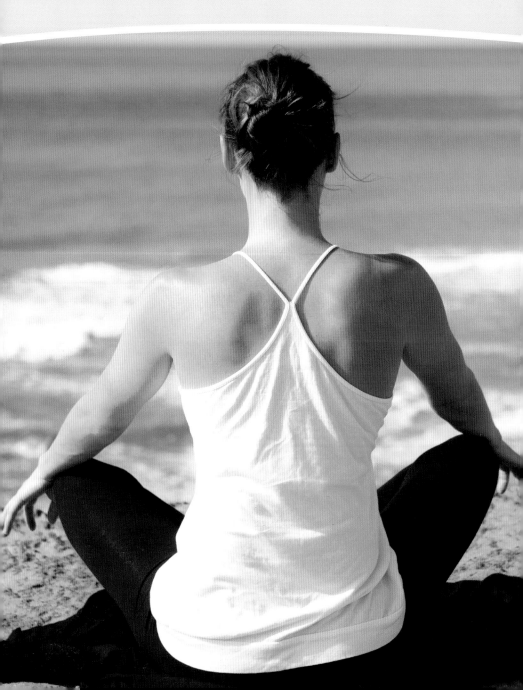

BACK

Back Exercises

The muscles of the back are another large muscle group that responds well to intensive training and heavier weights. A strong, firm back improves the body's posture and helps maintain overall health. However, many people ignore their back muscles or fail to exercise them when they work out.

Don't Forget Your Back!

The muscles of the back are crucial to health. They support your frame and your stomach muscles, or core. Having toned back muscles not only improves body shape and appearance, but also helps prevent the back pain and muscle strain that is commonly associated with people who have sedentary lifestyles.

Exercises for the Back

The following exercises will improve your posture and tighten and firm your back muscles. As with all the exercises in this book, begin with fewer repetitions until you are confident you are performing the exercise properly. Increase repetitions and weight as you progress with the exercises.

Back Goals

- **Improved posture**
- **Improved upper body strength**
- **Support for the core muscles**
- **Shapely rear physique**

Did You Know?

It is a good idea to try to focus on your posture, or form, when training your back to avoid strain and injury.

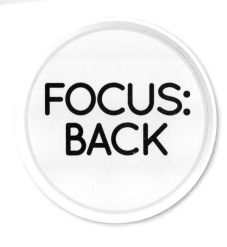

FOCUS: BACK

Single Arm Rows

- Position yourself on all fours
- With one hand, pick up your weight
- Raise the weight up towards the side of the chest, bending the elbow
- Keep the back flat and straight at all times
- Lower the weight to the floor
- Repeat equally on both arms

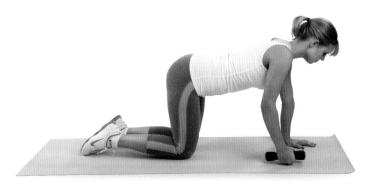

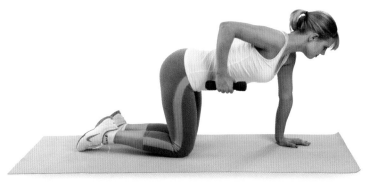

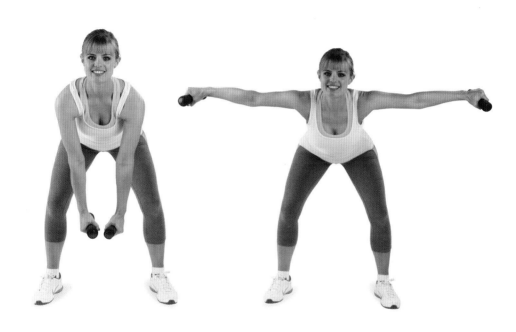

Back Fly

- Pick up your weights in both hands

- Stand with the feet shoulder-width apart, knees slightly bent

- Bend forwards, keeping the back flat and straight

- Keeping the arms straight, lift your weights directly out to the side of the body

- Controlling the movement, lower the weights, repeat

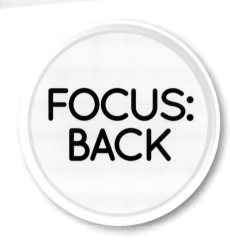

FOCUS:
BACK

Bentover Rows

- Pick up the weights in both hands

- Stand with the feet shoulder-width apart

- Bend forwards, keeping the back flat and straight. Hold the weights in front of you

- Bending the arms at the elbows, lift the weights up towards the chest, as if performing a rowing action

- Controlling the movement, return to starting position, repeat

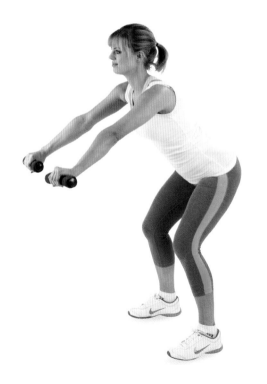

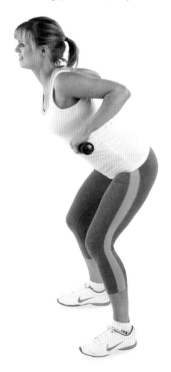

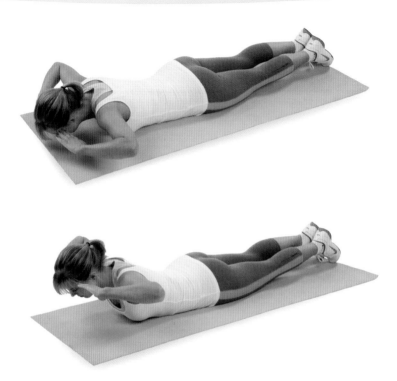

Back Raises

- Lie face down on the floor, with the fingertips touching the temples

- Slowly, raise the chest and upper back off the floor, looking straight down at the ground

- Lower yourself to the ground, back to the starting position and repeat

TRICEPS

Tricep Exercises

The tricep is a large muscle, but it is often underused. Triceps that are not worked regularly can result in the dreaded 'bingo wing' that many women complain about. The good news is that with consistent, targeted work it is possible to get the tricep muscle back into shape and looking good in sleeveless tops.

Targeted Training

Improving the muscle and tone of the triceps with targeted strength training exercises, will give the arms a better contour and also improve the texture and tone of the skin around the upper arm area. Women in particular tend to gather fat around the tricep area, however, combined with a healthy eating programme, exercise can help to target this problem area.

Your triceps may feel very weak when you first start to exercise them if you are unused to strength training. It is best to start with light weights and work up to heavier weights as you progress with your training. If you are committed and consistent with your training, you will start to notice a much improved tone to this muscle and soon get stronger and be able to lift heavier weights.

Cardio and Triceps

Certain cardio exercises are also good for tricep work; these include swimming and any other arm-focused activity, such as tennis, badminton and squash.

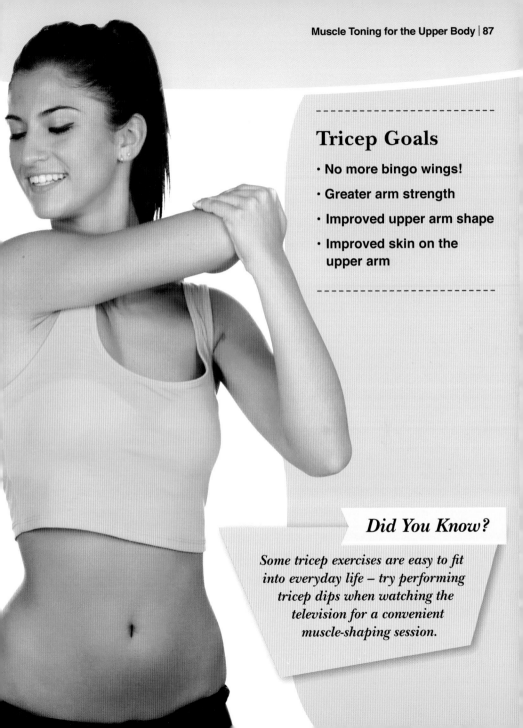

Tricep Goals

- **No more bingo wings!**
- **Greater arm strength**
- **Improved upper arm shape**
- **Improved skin on the upper arm**

Did You Know?

Some tricep exercises are easy to fit into everyday life – try performing tricep dips when watching the television for a convenient muscle-shaping session.

FOCUS: TRICEPS

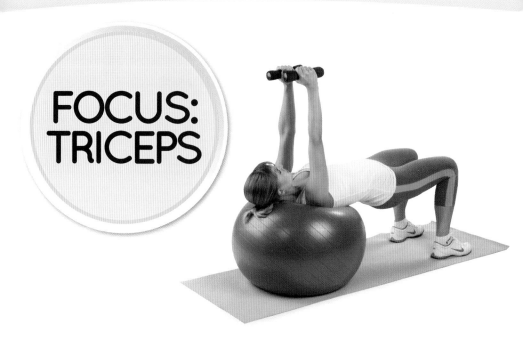

Skull Crushers

- Pick up the weights

- Lie on the back with the arms raised above the chest

- Slowly lower the weights until they are at either side of the forehead

- Slowly raise the weights again, controlling the movement. You should feel the exertion in the muscle at the back of the arms

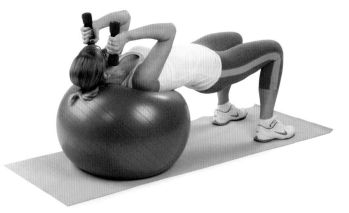

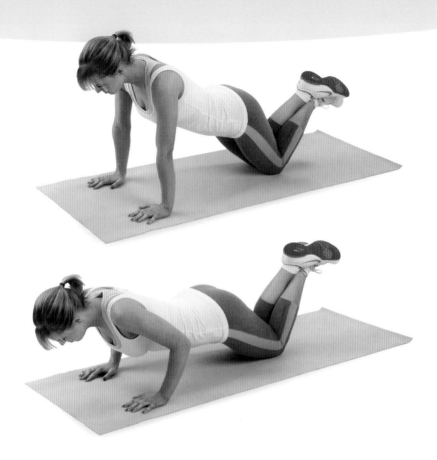

Tricep Press-ups

- Get into a press-up position, but with the hands shoulder-width apart. It is important that the arms are closer to the body, instead of the usual press-up position, in order to work the tricep muscles

- Slowly lower the chest towards the ground, hold the position for a few seconds

- Raise yourself to the starting position and repeat

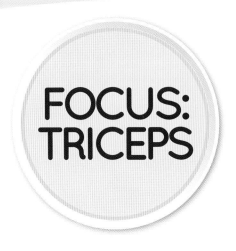

FOCUS: TRICEPS

Tricep Kickbacks

- Position yourself on all fours with a flat back

- Pick up a weight in one hand and raise so the arm is an L-shape and the tricep is in line with the back

- Slowly, extend the weight back, keeping the arm in line with the body, and straighten the arm

- Bend the elbow to return the weight back to the starting position, repeat

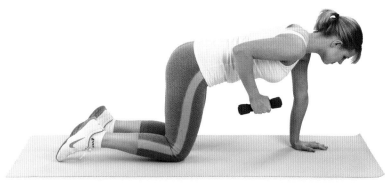

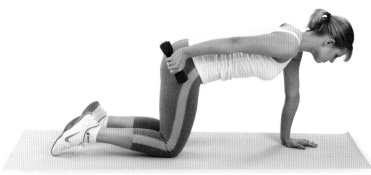

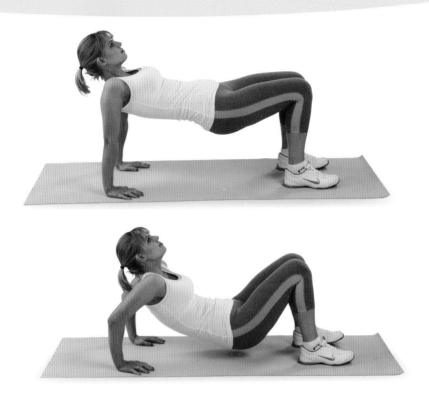

Tricep Dips

- Sit down with knees bent and feet positioned hip-width apart. Rest the hands on the ground behind, facing forward

- Lift the bottom off the ground, so that the back is parallel to the floor

- Dip down, bending the arms at the elbow, with the bottom an inch from the ground. Slowly return to starting position, repeat

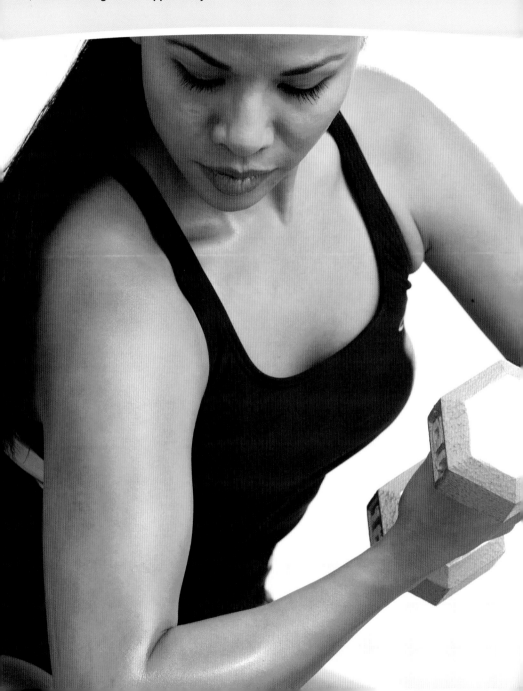

BICEPS

Bicep Exercises

The biceps are found at the front of the upper arm. This muscle is smaller than the triceps and generally easier to exercise. With consistent exercise, the biceps quickly respond to strength training and take on a firmer appearance. Exercising the biceps will result in a sculpted, toned upper arm and greater arm strength too.

The 'Guns'

Men who strength train often concentrate on working the bicep muscles which are also referred to as the 'guns'. Many women ignore their biceps when beginning a fitness programme, wrongly assuming this is a 'male-only' zone. Along with the triceps, working the biceps is the key to improving the appearance of the upper arm. Don't forget your biceps and remember to include them as part of your complete upper body workout.

Cardio Training and Strength

Focused strength training exercise targets this muscle. Running also activates the bicep muscle and can help improve its tone.

Bicep Goals

- **Defined upper arms**
- **Greater arm strength**
- **Improved tautness in the upper arm**

Did You Know?

By focusing on the bicep muscle as you train it, and noticing the contraction of the muscle, you'll avoid simply throwing the weight up and down.

FOCUS: BICEPS

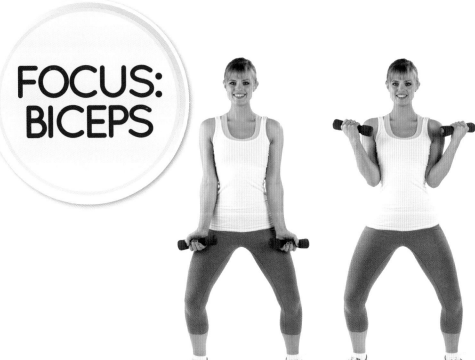

Bicep Curls

- Stand upright with knees bent and feet shoulder-width apart

- Hold your weights in each hand, arms resting on your thighs

- Slowly, pull the weights towards you, feeling the contraction of the biceps

- Lower the weights to thigh height, repeat

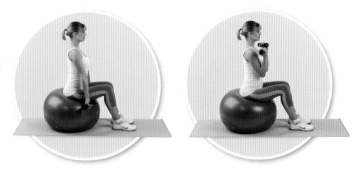

You can perform this exercise sitting or standing.

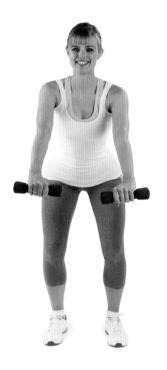 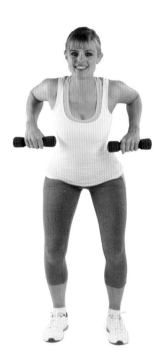

Bicep Pull-backs

- Stand upright, knees bent and feet shoulder-width apart

- Hold your weights in each hand, the arms held out in front of you at hip height

- Slowly, pull back the weights to chest height, feeling the contraction of the biceps. Lower the weights to hip height once more, repeat

- Lower the weights to hip height once more

SHOULDERS

Shoulder Exercises

The shoulder is a collection of muscles and tendons which require targeted work with a variety of exercises. The shoulder muscles are a 'ball-like' muscle group. Different exercises focus on the different parts of the shoulder.

Shapely Shoulders

Sculpting and shaping the shoulders is important to any fitness plan. The shoulders help define the body and balance the body. In men, developing the shoulders creates a V-shape physique, with a wider upper body and narrower waist. In women, defining the shoulders helps to balance the proportions of the body, making the waist and hips seem smaller. Women with a 'pear shape' physique often find that developing the shoulders improves the appearance of their body and can balance out wide hips and thighs, making them seem narrower in proportion to the upper body.

Targeted Toning

Cardio exercise such as running and swimming can also help firm and tone the shoulder muscles. Try to incorporate the strength training exercises on the following pages within your fitness routine for all over upper body strength and improved appearance.

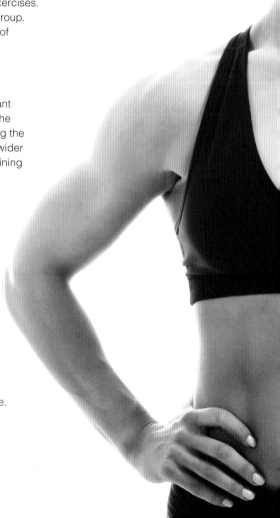

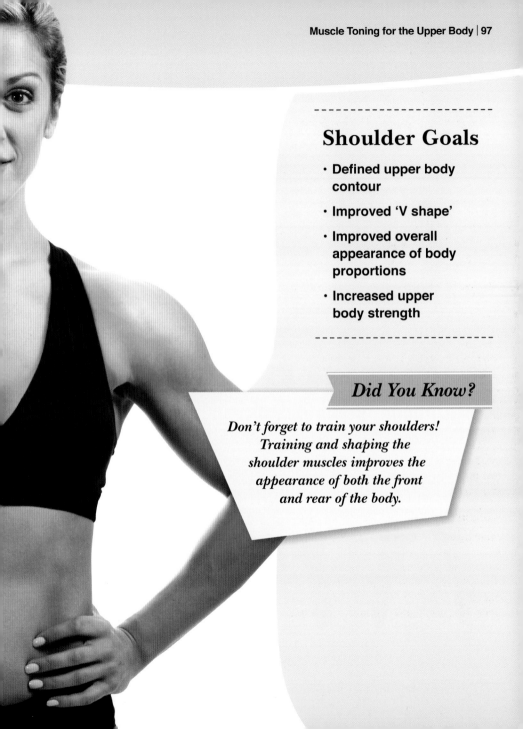

Shoulder Goals

- **Defined upper body contour**
- **Improved 'V shape'**
- **Improved overall appearance of body proportions**
- **Increased upper body strength**

Did You Know?

Don't forget to train your shoulders! Training and shaping the shoulder muscles improves the appearance of both the front and rear of the body.

FOCUS: SHOULDERS

Military Lift

- Stand upright, legs hip-width apart with the knees slightly bent. Hold your weights in both hands, in line with the shoulders

- Lift the weights up, extending the arm fully in line with the shoulders

- Feel the contraction in the shoulder muscles as you lift the weights

- Lower the weights to the starting position, repeat

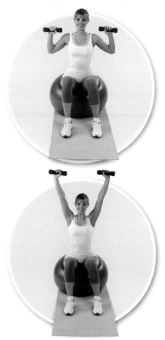

You can perform this exercise standing or sitting.

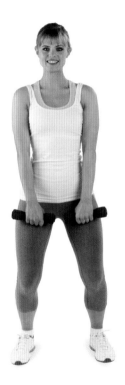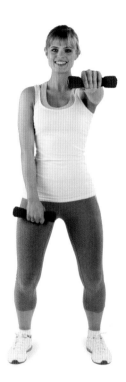

Front Lateral Raises

- Stand upright with the knees slightly bent and feet hip-width apart, holding the weights by the thighs

- Slowly, with a straight arm, extend one arm up and outwards to lift the weight to chest height

- Return the weight to the starting position and repeat

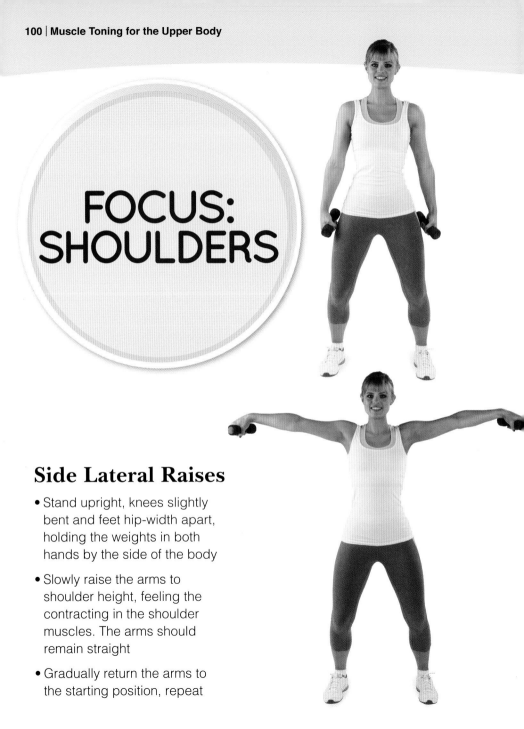

FOCUS: SHOULDERS

Side Lateral Raises

- Stand upright, knees slightly bent and feet hip-width apart, holding the weights in both hands by the side of the body

- Slowly raise the arms to shoulder height, feeling the contracting in the shoulder muscles. The arms should remain straight

- Gradually return the arms to the starting position, repeat

Back Lateral Raises

- Holding your weights in both hands with knees slightly bent and feet hip-width apart, bend forwards, keeping the back flat and straight

- Slowly extend the arms to the side of the body

- Return arms to starting position, repeat

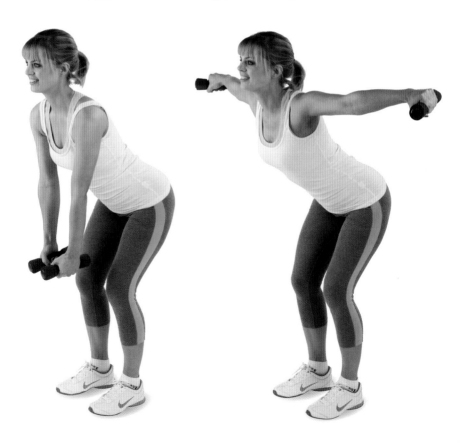

UPPER BODY Q&A

I have weak wrists, can I still strength train?

You should definitely strength train! Working with weights will improve your wrist strength, along with the rest of your upper body.

Isn't strength training for the upper body for men only?

Women often make the mistake of believing that upper body strength training is a male-only preserve. You'll often see women in a gym working hard on their lower body, but ignoring their upper body strength. The opposite is true of men! The key to a strong and shapely physique is balance – you need to work your upper body as well as your lower body to improve your overall shape and muscle definition. Never skip training your upper body.

Could I hurt myself if I try to lift heavy weights?

You should always start training with weights that feel comfortable for you – don't try to compete with anyone else. Remember, your goal is to slowly increase the heaviness of the weights that you lift. Injuries can occur if you move too quickly from a light weight to a heavy weight. If you monitor your progress, increase the weights slowly and carefully, and maintain your form at all times, you should be fine.

Won't I feel intimidated if I train my upper body at a gym?

A good gym will have respectful members and you should never be made to feel out of place. At first, it can feel intimidating to go to a gym, especially if you are unused to exercise or have not exercised for some time, but try to overcome these feelings by focusing on the end result. Remember, everyone at the gym is there for the same goal – to exercise and keep in shape.

If I work hard on my upper body strength training, can I eat what I like?

Diet is as crucial to achieving a great-looking and healthy body as is exercise – the two work hand in hand. Unless you supply your body with the nutrition it needs to repair and grow muscle, you will not achieve the results you desire. Likewise, overeating cannot be counteracted by exercising. Unless you are spending hours every day training intensively to the extent of an athlete, you'll need to watch your diet carefully.

My arms still look flabby despite training, what am I doing wrong?

Keep a diary to note your diet and training patterns. It may be that you are not training hard enough, or are overeating. Increase the intensity of your workouts and focus on your diet and cardio, too.

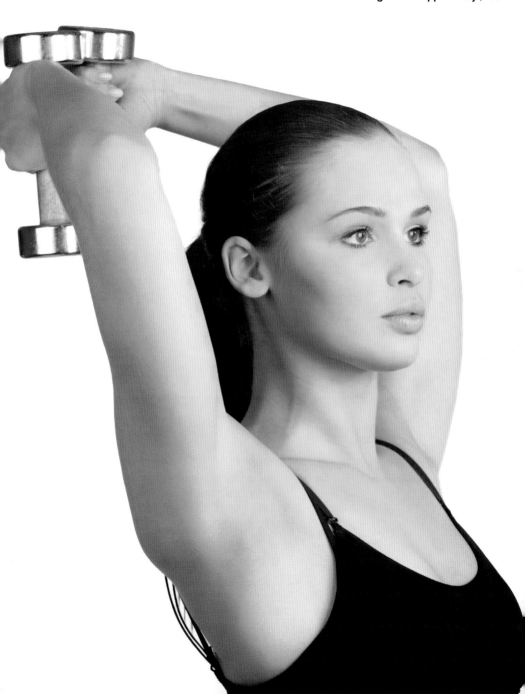

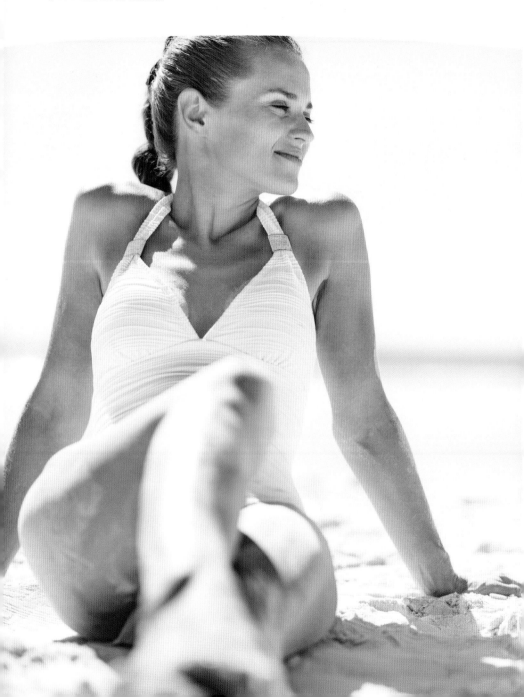

COUNTDOWN TO FITNESS

By this point, you should have all the information you need to establish an effective cardiovascular and strength training regimen. Now it's time to get your new exercise programme off to a great start. On the following pages you will find a 6-week fitness programme for a healthy and super-fit body!

Our easy-to-follow guide makes planning the first 6 weeks of your exercise simple and fuss-free. Follow the guides and gradually build up your stamina and muscle strength week by week. By week 6, you should see real results and be feeling fit, toned and healthy.

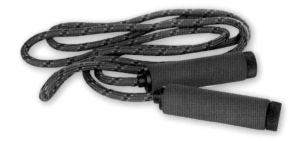

YOUR 6-WEEK PROGRAMME

This programme has been designed to get maximum results from your training. For beginners, you'll find a structured, safe routine. For regular exercisers, the programme will inject some life into an over-familiar routine and a tired training programme. To kick start your fitness goals, read and take note of the guidelines on the following pages.

Consistent Training

The programmes are based on consistent training over a 6-week period. They allow you to begin at a level that suits your current fitness and to assess your progress as you work through the course.

The training routines offer a mix of both cardiovascular exercise and strength training exercise to ensure that you cross-train, which is the best way to burn fat, tone up and increase your stamina. Remember, a mixture of strength training and cardiovascular workouts will rev up your metabolism and build muscle mass – which means you'll be burning more calories even while you watch the television. Try to ensure that you combine both forms of exercise to get the best results from your training.

Rest and Assess

After each training session, assess how your fitness levels are progressing.

Can you see an improvement in your stamina and speed? Are you starting to see improved skin and muscle tone? By regularly stepping back and assessing your progress, you will be able to stay focused on your individual goals and needs, and avoid simply 'going through the motions' with each training session.

Stay Focused

Try to approach each training session with a positive frame of mind and a determination to improve on your last exercise session. With a positive mental attitude, you'll be more likely to continue with the training programme and put in more effort with each session, thereby ensuring greater results.

Don't Give Up!

The most important thing is that you don't give up. If you find that some days you are tired or do not perform as well as you would have liked, simply start afresh the next day. Regular exercisers will tell you that your performance fluctuates, so don't beat yourself up if you have days when you don't train as well as others – the key is consistency and perseverance. Getting and keeping fit is for life!

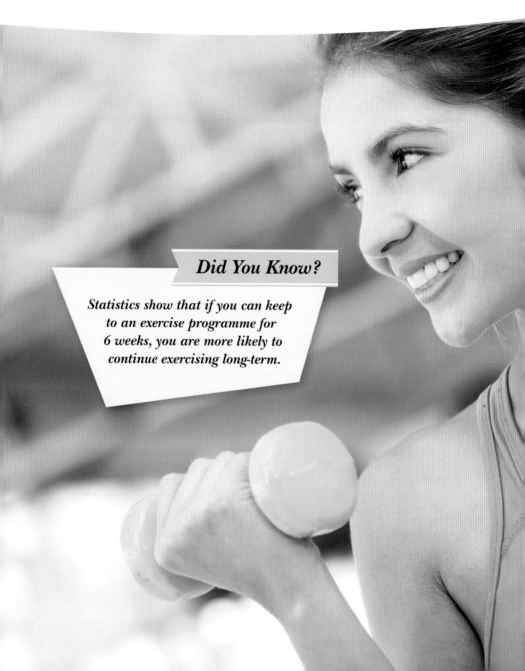

Did You Know?

Statistics show that if you can keep to an exercise programme for 6 weeks, you are more likely to continue exercising long-term.

GETTING STARTED

Aim to complete at least 3 cardio training sessions per week. You can increase this to 5 sessions, as long as you have time to complete them along with the strength training programmes. If you find 5 sessions are too much as you work through the 6-week programme, simply reduce the number of sessions as needed. You can select training routines from any of the running, cycling, swimming or class programmes outlined.

Cardio for Beginners and Intermediates

If you are new to exercise, keep to the beginner's programme for the duration of the first few weeks. If you are a regular exerciser, start with the beginner's programme and assess your fitness levels after your first couple of training sessions. If you are finding the routine too easy, go straight through to the intermediate sessions.

Cardio for Advanced Exercisers

If you exercise regularly, and to a relatively high intensity, begin with the intermediate session and if you find it too easy, move straight through to the advanced sessions.

Strength Training

Using the step-by-step exercises in the second section of this book, incorporate both targeted upper and lower body exercises in accordance with the guidelines in the 6-week charts.

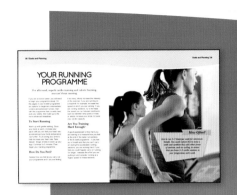

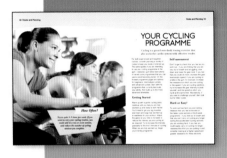

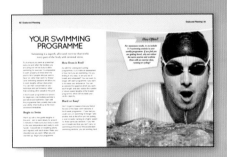

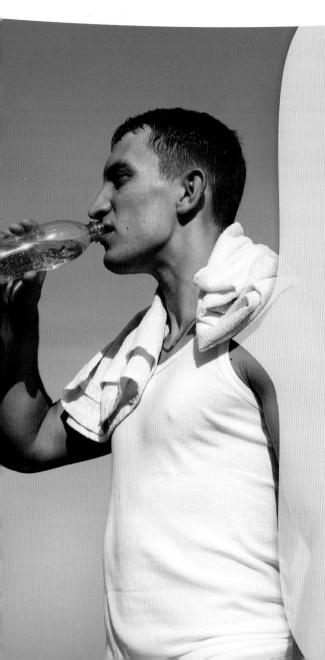

Preparation

Before you start your programme, it's worth running through a few key checklist points to make sure you are ready to get fit:

- -

A priority must be to ensure you have a comfortable pair of training shoes.

- -

Make sure you have exercise clothing you are comfortable in.

- -

Ensure you have all the equipment you need for your cardio and strength training sessions. Have you checked it is all in good working order?

- -

Wear a watch or carry a timer, so you can check the duration of your exercise sessions.

- -

Always take a bottle of water to each session and drink regularly to avoid becoming dehydrated.

- -

Plan the times at which you are going to exercise – avoid times when you are likely to be very tired or easily distracted.

- -

Keep your training programme in a visible place – it will remind you to exercise.

YOUR RUNNING PROGRAMME

Beginners:
15-minute programme

▌ Run moderately for
5 minutes

▌ Run quickly for
2 minutes

▌ Run moderately
for 2 minutes

▌ Run quickly for
2 minutes

▌ Run moderately for
2 minutes

▌ Run quickly for
2 minutes

▌ Run slowly for 1
minute to cool down

Intermediate Runners:
20-minute programme

▌ Run at a moderate speed
for 10 minutes

▌ Run at an accelerated
speed for 5 minutes –
you should find this speed
challenging

▌ Run at a moderate speed
for 5 minutes

▌ Run slowly for 1 minute to
cool down

Advanced Runners:
30-minute programme

▌ Run at a moderate speed for
5 minutes

▌ Run at a greatly accelerated
speed for 1 minute

▌ Run at a moderate speed for
4 minutes

▌ Run at a greatly accelerated
speed for 2 minutes

▌ Run at a moderate speed for
3 minutes

▌ Run at a greatly accelerated
speed for 3 minutes

▌ Run at a moderate speed for
2 minutes

▌ Run at a greatly accelerated
speed for 4 minutes

▌ Run at a moderate speed for
1 minute

▌ Run at a greatly accelerated
speed for 5 minutes

▌ Run slowly for 1 minute to
cool down

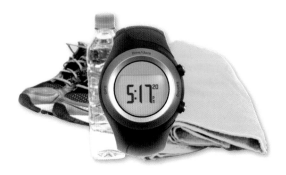

The levels on the programmes below indicate intensity if using a cycle machine in the gym.

YOUR CYCLING PROGRAMME

Beginners:
15-minute programme

- Cycle moderately for 2 minutes: level 4

- Cycle quickly for 2 minutes: level 5

- Cycle moderately for 3 minutes: level 4

- Cycle quickly for 2 minutes: level 5

- Cycle moderately for 3 minutes: level 4

- Cycle quickly for 3 minutes: level 5

- Cycle slowly for 1 minute to cool down

Intermediate Cyclists:
20-minute programme

- Cycle at a moderate speed for 3 minutes: level 4

- Cycle at an accelerated speed for 3 minutes: level 5

- Cycle at an intense speed for 3 minutes: level 6

- Cycle at an increasingly intense speed for 3 minutes: level 7

- Cycle at an intense speed for 3 minutes: level 6

- Cycle at an accelerated speed for 3 minutes: level 5

- Cycle at a moderate speed for 2 minutes: level 4

- Cycle slowly for 1 minute to cool down

Advanced Cyclists:
30-minute programme

- Cycle at a moderate speed for 3 minutes: level 4

- Cycle at an intense speed for 3 minutes: level 6

- Cycle at an accelerated speed for 3 minutes: level 5

- Cycle at an intense speed for 3 minutes: level 7

- Cycle at an accelerated speed for 3 minutes: level 6

- Cycle at maximum capacity for 2 minute: level 8

- Cycle at an intense speed for 3 minutes: level 6

- Cycle at an accelerated speed for 5 minutes: level 5

- Cycle at a moderate speed for 5 minutes: level 1

- Cycle slowly for 1 minute to cool down

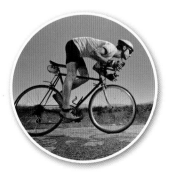

YOUR SWIMMING PROGRAMME

Beginners:
15-minute programme

▎ Swim at a steady pace for 4 lengths

▎ Swim at an accelerated pace for 2 lengths

▎ Continue for the duration of a 15-minute workout

▎ Cool down with 1 minute of gentle swimming

Intermediate Swimmers:
20-minute programme

▎ Swim at a steady pace for 4 lengths

▎ Swim at an accelerated pace for 2 lengths

▎ Swim at a steady pace for 4 lengths

▎ Swim at an accelerated pace for 3 lengths

▎ Swim at a steady pace for 4 lengths

▎ Swim at an accelerated pace for 4 lengths

▎ Continue for the duration of a 20-minute workout

▎ Cool down with 1 minute of gentle swimming

Advanced Swimmers:
30-minute programme

▎ Swim at a steady pace for 3 lengths

▎ Swim at an accelerated pace for 1 length

▎ Swim at a steady pace for 2 lengths

▎ Swim at an accelerated pace for 2 lengths

▎ Swim at a steady pace for 1 length

▎ Swim at an accelerated pace for 3 lengths

▎ Swim at a steady pace for 1 length

▎ Swim at an accelerated pace for 4 lengths

▎ Continue for the duration of a 30-minute workout

▎ Cool down with 1 minute of gentle swimming

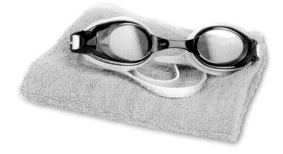

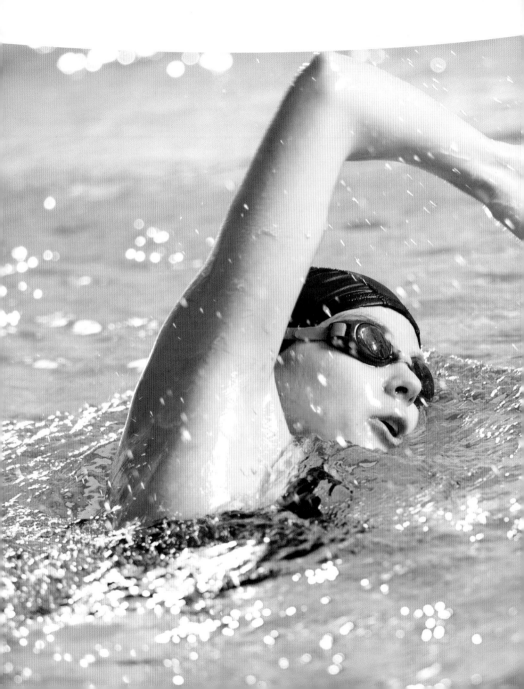

YOUR PROGRAMME
WEEK 1

Day
1

Cardio Training
15–30 minutes cardio training

Day
2

Strength Training
15 minutes upper body exercises to include:
Chest • Back • Biceps and Triceps • Core

Day
3

Cardio Training
15–30 minutes cardio training

Day
4

Rest Day
Allow your body to recover

Day
5

Strength Training
15 minutes lower body and shoulder
exercises to include: Buttocks • Legs
• Shoulders • Core

Day
6

Cardio Training
15–30 minutes cardio training

Day
7

Rest Day
Allow your body to recover

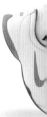

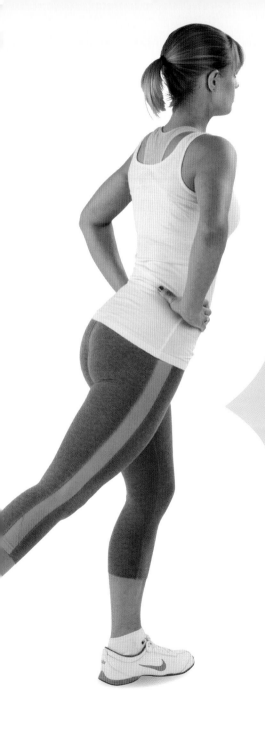

Cardio Goals

- Beginners should keep to just 15 minutes per session for week 1.

- Intermediates should aim to complete 20 minutes per session for week 1.

- Advanced exercisers should aim to complete 30 minutes per session for week 1.

Strength Training Goals

- Beginners should keep to just 5 repetitions per exercise for week 1.

- Intermediates should aim for 10 repetitions per exercise for week 1.

- Advanced exercisers should aim for 15 repetitions per exercise for week 1, gradually increasing weight.

YOUR PROGRAMME
WEEK 2

Day
1

Cardio Training
15–35 minutes cardio training

Day
2

Strength Training
20 minutes upper body exercises to include:
Chest • Back • Biceps and Triceps • Core

Day
3

Cardio Training
15–35 minutes cardio training

Day
4

Rest Day
Allow your body to recover

Day
5

Strength Training
20 minutes lower body and shoulder exercises to
include: Buttocks • Legs • Shoulders • Core

Day
6

Cardio Training
15–35 minutes cardio training

Day
7

Rest Day
Allow your body to recover

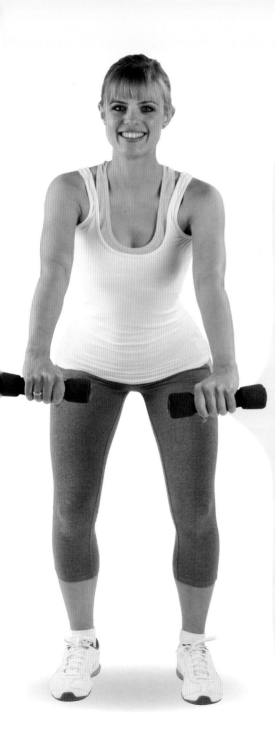

Cardio Goals

- Beginners should keep to just 15–20 minutes per session for week 2.

- Intermediates should aim to complete 20–25 minutes per session for week 2.

- Advanced exercisers should aim to complete 30–35 minutes per session for week 2.

Strength Training Goals

- Beginners should aim for 5 repetitions per exercise for week 2.

- Intermediates should aim for 10 repetitions per exercise for week 2.

- Advanced exercisers should aim for 15 repetitions per exercise for week 2 gradually increasing weight.

YOUR PROGRAMME
WEEK 3

Day 1

Cardio Training
20–40 minutes cardio training

Day 2

Strength Training
25 minutes upper body exercises to include:
Chest • Back • Biceps and Triceps • Core

Day 3

Cardio Training
20–40 minutes cardio training

Day 4

Rest Day
Allow your body to recover

Day 5

Strength Training
25 minutes lower body and shoulder exercises to include: Buttocks • Legs • Shoulders • Core

Day 6

Cardio Training
20–40 minutes cardio training

Day 7

Cardio Training or Rest Day
20–40 minutes cardio training, or rest depending on your fitness levels at this stage

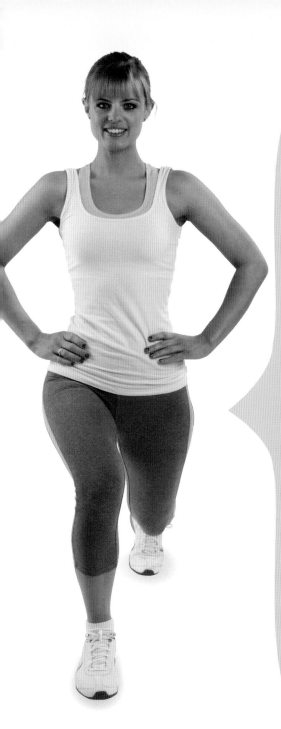

Cardio Goals

- Beginners should keep to just 20–25 minutes per session for week 3.

- Intermediates should aim to complete 30–35 minutes per session for week 3.

- Advanced exercisers should aim to complete 40 minutes per session for week 3.

Strength Training Goals

- Beginners should aim for 5–7 repetitions per exercise for week 3.

- Intermediates should aim for 10–12 repetitions per exercise for week 3.

- Advanced exercisers should aim for 15 repetitions per exercise for week 3, gradually increasing weight.

YOUR PROGRAMME WEEK 4

Day 1

Cardio Training
20–45 minutes cardio training

Day 2

Strength Training
35 minutes upper body exercises to include:
Chest • Back • Biceps and Triceps • Core

Day 3

Cardio Training
20–45 minutes cardio training

Day 4

Rest Day
Allow your body to recover

Day 5

Strength Training
35 minutes lower body and shoulder exercises to
include: Buttocks • Legs • Shoulders • Core

Day 6

Cardio Training
20–45 minutes cardio training

Day 7

Strength Training
35 minutes full body exercises to include: Buttocks
Legs • Shoulders • Triceps and Biceps • Core

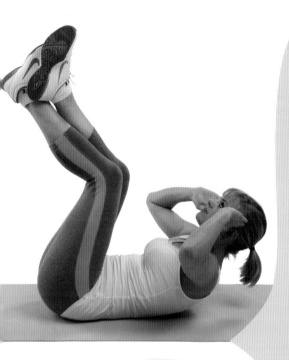

Cardio Goals

- Beginners should keep to 20–25 minutes per session for week 4.

- Intermediates should aim to complete 30–35 minutes per session for week 4.

- Advanced exercisers should aim to complete 40–45 minutes per session for week 4.

Strength Training Goals

- Beginners should aim for 7–10 repetitions per exercise for week 4.

- Intermediates should aim for 12–15 repetitions per exercise for week 4.

- Advanced exercisers should aim for 15 repetitions per exercise for week 4, gradually increasing weight.

Rest and Assess

Stay focused on the level of intensity you are working to in each session. Could you work harder or are you training at a pace you can't maintain? Adjust week by week to suit your progression and individual needs.

YOUR PROGRAMME
WEEK 5

Day 1

Cardio Training
30–50 minutes cardio training

Day 2

Strength Training
40 minutes upper body exercises to include:
Chest • Back • Biceps and Triceps • Core

Day 3

Cardio Training
30–50 minutes cardio training

Day 4

Rest Day
Allow your body to recover

Day 5

Strength Training
40 minutes lower body and shoulder exercises to
include: Buttocks • Legs • Shoulders • Core

Day 6

Cardio Training
30–50 minutes cardio training

Day 7

Strength Training
40 minutes full body exercises to include: Buttocks
Legs • Shoulders • Triceps and Biceps • Core

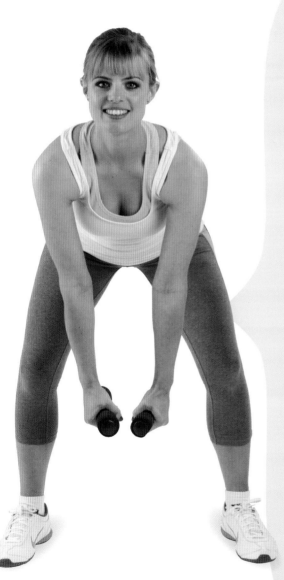

Cardio Goals

- Beginners should keep to 30–35 minutes per session for week 5.

- Intermediates should aim to complete 35–45 minutes per session for week 5.

- Advanced exercisers should aim to complete 50 minutes per session for week 5.

Strength Training Goals

- Beginners should aim for 10–12 repetitions per exercise for week 5.

- Intermediates should aim for 15 repetitions per exercise for week 5. Start to increase the weights at this stage.

- Advanced exercisers should aim for 15 repetitions per exercise for week 5. Increase the weights if needed.

YOUR PROGRAMME
WEEK 6

Day 1

Cardio Training
35–60 minutes cardio training

Day 2

Strength Training
40 minutes upper body exercises to include:
Chest • Back • Biceps and Triceps • Core

Day 3

Cardio Training
35–60 minutes cardio training

Day 4

Rest Day
Allow your body to recover

Day 5

Strength Training
40 minutes lower body and shoulder exercises to
include: Buttocks • Legs • Shoulders • Core

Day 6

Cardio Training
35–60 minutes cardio training

Day 7

Strength Training
40 minutes full body exercises to include: Buttocks •
Legs • Shoulders • Triceps and Biceps • Core

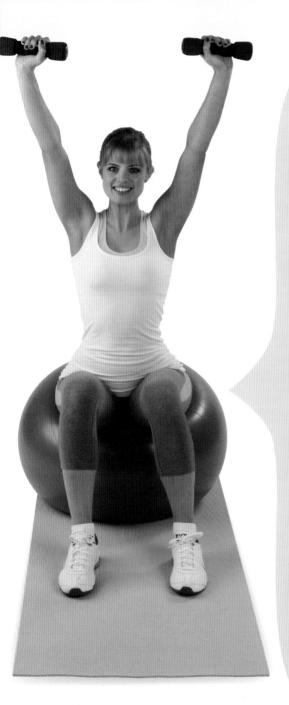

Cardio Goals

- Beginners should keep to 35–40 minutes per session for week 6.
- Intermediates should aim to complete 45–50 minutes per session for week 6.
- Advanced exercisers should aim to complete 60 minutes per session for week 6.

Strength Training Goals

- Beginners should aim for 12 repetitions per exercise for week 6.
- Intermediates should aim for 15 repetitions per exercise for week 6, using heavier weights.
- Advanced exercisers should aim for 15 repetitions per exercise for week 6, with increased weights.

GLOSSARY

abdominals the stomach muscles

arm rotations moving the arm in a circular pattern to loosen the shoulder joint and warm up the upper body

barbell a piece of equipment used in weight training. A barbell is made up of a long bar to which circular weights are fixed

bicep the muscle at the front of the arm

body mass index (BMI) calculation using height and weight to assess if a person is within their optimum weight range

cardio capacity the rate at which the heart can pump blood around the body

cardiovascular exercise that increases the heart rate and the intake and circulation of oxygen around the body

cellulite unsightly fat around the thighs, stomach and arms. Cellulite gives the skin a wrinkled and uneven appearance

circulation the pumping of blood around the body

combat classes exercise classes that use fighting techniques such as boxing movements

core the muscles of the stomach

cross-country across open countryside

cross-train to build a mixture of exercise forms into a routine, such as strength training and cardiovascular exercise

dehydrated a condition in which the body does not have enough water. Dehydration is caused by not drinking enough water

dumbbells hand-held weights

elasticity the ability to bounce back; skin that has elasticity does not sag

endorphin a hormone that improves a person's mood, making him or her feel happier

gluteus maximus the muscle of the buttock

intensity the level of ease or effort with which exercise is performed

intermediate the stage between a novice and an experienced exerciser

ligaments tissues that support and connect muscle to bone

metabolic rate the speed at which the body burns calories

motivation the desire to do something, such as exercise

muscle group a particular area of muscle, such as the chest muscles or the back muscles

muscle mass the density and size of muscle

obliques the muscles that run down the side of the body from the rib cage to the hips

optimum body fat a level of body fat that is neither underweight nor overweight

overdeveloped muscle that has been overtrained so that it is no longer in proportion

posture the way that a person stands and holds his or her body

repetitions the number of times an exercise is performed, such as lunge repetitions or bicep curl repetitions

resistance the force that a person works against when performing an exercise

sedentary lifestyle a lifestyle in which daily life involves mainly sitting and not moving around a great deal

stamina the ability to perform exercise for a sustained period

static machines resistance machines found in gyms on which the user can strength train. Static machines are fixed in position, unlike free weights such as dumbbells or barbells

stationary bike a bike located in a gym, or sold for home use, that is fixed in position

strength training exercise that focuses on increasing muscle mass and capacity, such as weight training

sustained activity exercise that is continuous and unbroken for a period of time

technique the way in which an exercise is performed

tendons tissues that support and connect muscle and bone

testosterone a hormone that allows the body to build muscle, plus other fuctions. Testosterone levels are higher in men than in women

tricep the muscle at the back of the arm

trunk the central part of the body consisting of the chest, back and stomach area

INDEX